Rocko

MW01125718

Dr.Shawn Baker
The carnivore diet: Evolution, lessons & implementation

———

How you can improve your health with an animal & science based nutrition - featuring Tom Bilyeu.

———

Revised Transcripts

25% of the royalties will go to Dr. Thomas Seyfrieds cancer research! See KetoforCancer.net

P.S.: Any review would be GREATLY appreciated to get the Low-Carb message out!

TABLE OF CONTENTS

.

Chapter 1
The Evolutionary Logic Behind the Carnivore Diet - Shawn Baker on Health Theory

Host Tom Bilyeu:

Hi everyone! Welcome to *Health Theory*. Today's guest is Dr. Shawn Baker.

He's an orthopedic surgeon, record-setting powerlifter, one-time semi-professional rugby player, all-american track and field masters athlete, former nuclear weapons launch officer - and most recently, the guy known for popularizing the carnivore diet!

Shawn, that's where I want to start. The carnivore diet obviously has gotten a little bit controversial. People are kind of weird about it. I'll say, I do what I call a *lazy man's carnivore diet*. So probably 90% of my calories come from meats, primarily red meat and some pork.

What is it that makes a carnivore diet so controversial - and why do you still think it's worth trying?

Dr. Shawn Baker:

First of all Tom, thanks for having me on. The carnivore diet certainly is controversial because it goes against what we've been told, from a nutrition science standpoint, for the last hundred years or so.

If we tell people that meat is really bad for us - particularly red meat - we've heard that for decades now. But we've got people that are really only eating red meat. And what you would expect to happen to their health is: They would get very sick acutely, or even over a period of time.

But in fact, what we're seeing is quite the opposite! That is something that rubs a lot of people the wrong way because they have a lot of personal investment in a different narrative. And I think that is why it's partially controversial.

There's a sort of a comfort in saying *everything in moderation*, in balance - even though we can't really accurately define even what that means, quite honestly. But

3

that's just sort of a platitude... people put out "Well, I believe in a balanced diet."

When I ask people "What does that mean to you? And what does it mean to somebody from another culture?" - those people have very different definitions. So we have to look at the full spectrum of human existence, to say what is the ideal diet.

And as humans, we're very lucky that we have a diverse capacity to eat a lot of different things. I would say that if you were to take people from 100,000 years ago and offer them Doritos and Twinkies, they would definitely eat them. But that does not mean we're designed for that!

Bilyeu:
That's really interesting to me. Are there things, cues, that we can look at humans to see if we're a true omnivore... and what does that mean?

Dr. Baker:
There's no doubt that humans are omnivorous. I mean, we clearly are! We can look at every human that has been on the planet, we could say that they've been eating a little bit of everything. The question is *how much of what* is represented.

So when we look at how to determine what something is suited for, really as a human being, these things are important:

What is the overall impact to your health, to your performance, to how you feel subjectively and objectively? Meaning, you feed somebody a certain diet and see what happens to them.

I would say that if you're eating the wrong diet, things probably occur that shouldn't occur. I think most disease that we see today has in some part a dietary component!

If we sit there and eat this modern industrial diet of novel foods that really aren't designed for us, we see what happens. We see depression, we see autoimmune disease, we see

4

gastrointestinal problems, we see chronic obesity. We see all these things.

A lot of these things we tribute to aging - which probably aren't really aging, it's just disease! I like to use...

The world record for a 100 meters sprint at 85 is about 15 seconds.

Bilyeu:
At 85 years old?

Dr. Baker:
85 years old, which is a pretty decent time. So I like to say "If you could run a 100 meters in 15 seconds, you're probably on the right side of being dead."

This is just a simple heuristic but it makes sense, you know. Think about a wild animal: The weak, the slow get eaten. Right? The same thing happens to humans: As we break down, as we deteriorate... we don't get eaten by lions, we get eaten by disease.

So if you can maintain, you know, whatever you were at, say 25... whenever you were at your physical peak and you can stay as close to that as possible, for as long as possible - you've not only prolonged your life, but most importantly, prolonged the quality of your life. Prolonged your functionaliy.

And there's clear evidence that athletic ability, lean muscle mass, protects you from disease. It protects you from dying, it allows you to function better. I think it can be as simple as that.

Bilyeu:
How old are you ?

Dr. Baker:
53

Bilyeu:

Okay. Talking about holding peak performance as you age: I know last year, you set a rowing record and you're going back to defend that again. That's certainly very impressive.

How do you maintain that peak level of performance?

Dr. Baker:

Well, just to be accurate: I won a world championship last year. I set three World Records when I turned 50. When I was at the World Championship, I was in the 50+ plus age class.

I've been training my whole life. It's not like one day I woke up and said "Ha! I'm gonna be a good athlete!" I've been consistently doing the basics for 40+ years, and it's something that's important to me. I'm a competitive guy, it drives me. It's part of my identity, it's kind of just built in at this point.

But I eat what I think is a very good diet... and I'm not promoting that everybody needs to do a carnivorous diet!

Bilyeu:

Do you back off that because there's so much backlash around? Or do you back off of that because truly, truly, it won't work for some people?

Dr. Baker:

No, I back off because I think most people don't need to do it. I mean, there's people that are doing largely well above average, very good from a health perspective. And if they're doing great, I don't see what you need to change it for.

Bilyeu:

Is the metric they use... because - at least in the interviews that I heard with you- you don't worry about your blood levels.

So, is it that you just go "Hey, how do you feel? How do you perform?" - and that's the metric you should care about?

Dr. Baker:

Let me clarify: It's not that I don't agree with blood tests or that I haven't checked them! Because I've done a round of blood test because people were asking me. I was like "Okay, I'll just do it. No big deal."

But you have to be very careful in your interpretation of blood tests because you have to put it in clinical context. As a physician, I viewed thousands upon thousands of blood tests.

And very often, you'll get one that's not quite perfectly within a standard reference range. Then, you'll say "Is that relevant to what's going on with that particular patient?"

So we have a lot of people that are kind of armchair quarterbacks, trying to do medicine with lab work - and they just look at these labs and say "Aha! That one's out of range, you must be sick!" - and that's not necessarily true.

We have to understand that many of these labs have incredible variability. Cholesterol is one of these things. A guy named David Feldman has shown that you can change your LDL cholesterol 100 points in three or four days!

And so, you go once a year for your annual test and your cholesterol is borderline high... and your doctor says "Hey, we're going to put you on this drug for the rest of your life!" - when you could have come in three days later and it would have been normal!

Your blood level of Vitamin D can change 30% in a day, within the course of a day, depending on what time of day you get it drawn. Things like cholesterol, all these other ones, they change so much.

So what you really want to know is what is going on chronically.

Things like a *coronary artery calcium scan:* That's a cardiac test you can take, looking at the calcium in your heart. It gives you an idea...

Bilyeu:

How do run that test?

Dr. Baker:
It's a CT scan. I had that done about two years into the diet
- and *my coronary calcium is a perfect zero!* No
calcification! That is a very good metric for assessing disease.

Now, there are people saying "Well, it might miss
plaques," and so on and so forth. But still, the people that
have no calcium have the least likelihood of having plaque
or anything from cardiovascular disease.

An easy method is just waist to height measurement: We
know that if your belly is too big, relative to your height,
you're at risk for metabolic problems... you basically have
metabolic disease.

These things that are more accurate chronic
representations. Because there's a lot of people out there
walking around that have really nice lab values, but they're
not healthy. The problem is: When we chase lab values,
rather than health, we get a very different set of goals.

Somebody could have a perfectly stable blood glucose for
ten years and they have hyperinsulinemia, in the
background. They have disease, they have the
pathophysiology going on - but we just haven't detected it
yet! So I think that's a bit of a travesty, quite honestly.

Bilyeu:
So breaking out of that, though: What should people be
paying attention to? Things I've heard you say before...

Okay, we've got waist to height ratio. You've got... if you're
a guy, are you waking up with erections. You've got the
calcification of the heart.

What are other things that we should really pay attention
to?

Dr. Baker:
I think insulin sensitivity is probably a useful metric. If you
look at the relationship of pretty much every chronic disease
and hyperinsulinemia, we see a pretty consistent

8

relationship. Now, again, I sort of rally against associations because there's some problems with that.

But in general, those things are important. Like I said... you mentioned sexual function. That's very important. I mean, some people laugh about it, but it's a very important part of health.

Bilyeu:
Why is it important? I've heard... it's said tha erectile dysfunction is a precursor to heart disease. Like, if you're having vascular problems there, chances are that you have a bigger problem going on at the level of the heart.

Dr. Baker:
Yeah, absolutely. Some people call it the canary in the coalmine. And, obviously, the male sex organ is a blood dependent organ! So when you do have impeded blood flow in any part of your body, it's probably occurring systemically - unless there's some trauma or something like that.

We see that, it is a concern for cardiovascular disease. So the fact that, at 53 years of age, I wake up every day with an erection - that indicates what's going on with my heart. Because, as I said, I had a coronary calcium scan of zero.

And: What I'm doing athletically would also indicate good cardiovascular function.

I don't know if you've ever been on one of these... if you've been to CrossFit or something like that, with the Concept 2 rowing machine - these are very challenging, from a cardiovascular standpoint.

Bilyeu:
That's interesting. Talk to me about exercise, heart health. Obviously you're very known for talking about diet. But also... I mean, just standing next to you: You are a wall of muscle! So you clearly take care of yourself, physically. You push yourself.

Like you said, that people look at aging is sort of this inevitable thing. But in reality, you've retained a lot of muscle mass. So

1) Can we add muscle as we age?
2) Why does that matter? And then,
3) How do we do it?

Dr. Baker:
Yes. As far as "Can you gain muscle?" - yes, you can definitely gain muscle pretty much at any age. There's studies in people in their 70s, in their 80s, showing they can put on muscle mass.

Now, the formula for that is pretty simple. It's adequate protein, adequate leucine, resistance training - either heavy weight or light weight. You've got to stimulate the muscles maximally.

And then, for many people, it's some sort of caloric surplus. You can get that through carbohydrates, you can get that through fat.

But beyond that, what do you have to do? I mean, at this point at 53, I like to make sure that I spend some time dedicated to actually getting stronger. That is basic compound movements. Also, some time spent trying to build muscle, to maintain that.

It's not that you have to have huge giant bodybuilder muscles. But having lean muscle mass, being in the top... There's a nice study, the *Honolulu Longevity Study,* that looked at strength in midlife:

People that were in the highest quartile for strength had a 250% chance increase of making it to 100 years of age.
Bilyeu:
Whoa!

Dr. Baker:
It's so important to do that, it's almost as important as genetics!

10

Bilyeu:
What... is it muscle mass, muscle density? The ability to contract the muscle? Because I've heard you say *it's not necessarily size. it's strength.*

Dr. Baker:
Yeah.

Bilyeu:
Is it that in the study, they didn't make a differentiation between strength and size? Because if I really think at just a biological level what's going on, it would seem like:

If you get really sick, there are amino acids and things you're gonna go down and strip from your own muscle, to recover from that - and if you have no muscle to strip, then you're just done.

But that would lead me to believe that size would be pretty important...?

Dr. Baker:
Yes, so there's a clear correlation between cross-sectional muscle area and strength. But sometimes, that's being challenged, some research is showing that you can be very strong with relatively smaller muscles.

So I think ultimately, when we look at longevity, it's really strength... and really *strength to size ratio,* that's important. So you want to be lean and strong.

And with strength comes function! Function is very important. When we lose some of our independence for walking. Again, when we get to the end of life, we see people that lose some independence with walking - and strength says plays a big role in that.

It's not that there's no relationship between strength and size. There is some, but the research has shown that strength is the more important factor for longevity and aging.

Quite honestly: Because most of us look at older people, older people are typically not bodybuilders. So we're not looking at *Mr. Olympia versus the the puny guy,* we're looking at normal people, a normal distribution...

With those normal people we can say "Of these kind of normal people, the ones that are on the stronger end of the spectrum do better than the people that aren't."

When you don't have much physiologic reserve, particularly muscle mass... when we do get struck with disease, cancer, infectious disease, something like that - not having that sort of buffer that the muscle provides tends to produce a worse outcome.

Bilyeu:
Yeah, that's super interesting. I want to go back and walk through the lineage of how humans ended up here. So the evolution question.

One day I was thinking "Okay, where do we fall in the spectrum of what we should be eating?" - and all of that. And I was like "Alright, if we share a common ancestor with monkeys and chimpanzees, gorillas, whatever... Obviously, gorillas chew a ton. Like, they're all about leaves."

I know that chimpanzees actually get some percentage of their calories from killing other animals... not the least of which being other chimpanzees.

So how much do you think is there truth to 'We came down out of the trees as food became more scarce. As we started turning into hunters, we find cooking,' all of that stuff that allows us to grow the bigger brain.

What was that rough step-by-step process, that you think led us to being the omnivores that we are?

Dr. Baker:
Yeah. So if we go back even further, there's research now that shows that the very first animals, the very first multicellular animals, started out as carnivorous animals.

When you think about it: When you're trying to build a structure it's very easy to take like and build like. So when we go to a different sort of building materials, it becomes less efficient. You have to have specialized adaptations.

Going back about 800 million years, the very first animals appear to be carnivore. And most of the animals that have ever been on the planet have been carnivorous. So: An herbivore is a really specialized adaptation!

Grasslands evolved about a hundred million years ago, so we started seeing the first larger herbivores come in then,

But if we go back to primate evolution, about 20 million years, we've had monkeys and eventually the ones that are still remaining, the bonobos, the chimpanzees, the gorillas... they've had 25 million years of evolution to try and develop increased brain size - and they've been doing it on a fruit based diet.

It has not worked! You've got 25 million years to try - and it doesn't work! So something had to change, to allow the differentiation into what we are now.

If we look back on the global climate record, starting between five and three million years ago, we saw a dramatic shift in what happened with global temperatures. We went from a lush tropical environment to a very much colder, a savanna type of situation, grasslands.

If we look at what people, humans and pre humans, were experiencing: It was more kind of Canada and not Costa Rica! We've got this situation where the food supply is very different.

And some of the early hominids tried to make it on a vegetarian diet. There are things like *Australopithecus Robustus* - and they just went extinct! Because they couldn't survive in the environment.

So we've had... in human evolution, all kinds of humans evolved. And what occurred was: As we grew this bigger brain, it required a more and more efficient, effective caloric dense fuel source - and that was animal fat!

And we know, going back to *Homo Erectus*, just with simple spear technology, they had no trouble killing elephants! That's what they usually hunted, that was their their food of choice.

Think about it: If you and I were to be magically transported back 50,000 years and our technology was spears - we could say "Well, you can gather plants for three days to get 1000, 2000 calories. Or you can go out and kill one of these big slow things, that doesn't run away, that just looks at you."

Because, remember: These animals sort of evolved with really no predators. I mean, Lions might eat the small elephants. But beyond that, once they're full size, they're like "What are you going to do to me, cute little human?"

So those early hunters had this abundance of food, abundance of fuel, that helped them to grow that bigger brain. I think that's what occured.

Also, comparative anatomy: If you look at another primate and we look at their digestive tract.

Humans have, on an anatomic basis... looking at what the hardware does, not the software. But the hardware. Seventeen percent of our digestive tract is able to ferment.

When we compare that to a chimp, an ape or an gorilla, they've got something like 50 to 60 percent of their gut, that can ferment.

So we lost much of that fermentative capacity - which means we cannot get a lot of nutrition from fiber or leaves. They eat leaves. We can't get much nutrition from that.

That's one of the reasons why a plant-based diet helps people lose weight because they're just not absorbing much nutrition - so they lose weight. Maybe it's not the best way to lose weight. So we just don't have that capacity anymore.

Bilyeu:
It's really interesting! Now, given that we have this 17% ability to ferment: When you hear the standard advice about "All things in moderation"... like, there's something intuitive about that, that feels right. Still, I've never lived my life like that.

But when people say it, I'm always like "Oh God" - there is something haunting about that.

And if we know that we are omnivores, why is it advantageous to go so full into carnivore? Is there something that's missed, is it a complete diet? Could you literally live on red meat forever?

Or are there times where you feel that it's important to dip in and out, have some vegetables... because there are micronutrients or whatever missing?

Dr. Baker:
Yes. So if you were to ask me what is probably a realistic ancient diet for humans, it's probably a whole bunch of meat and a few plants here and there. Probably fruit being the most common.

If you think about what's available to us? Fruit is generally well tolerated. But: Nuts and seeds without processing can be very... you know, a handful of cashews raw can kill you. Five kidney beans can kill you! If you eat them unprocessed. That was probably the basic diet.

Now, we have so many people today where their digestive system has probably been destroyed by, I think, seed oils - and some of these other products that they were exposed to.

I think that compromises people so they don't tolerate other foods

Bilyeu:
Why do you think seed oil is the big problem?

Dr. Baker:
There is some researchers, a group out of Hungary called the Paleomedicina group. And they've looked at gut permeability and there's something that's called *leaky gut*.

Normally, our digestive tract... we eat the food, we absorb the things we want to take in - and we don't allow anything else extra to come in. There is some degree of permeability that's normal.

But we get this exaggerated permeability that occurs when we're exposed to certain foods. Seed oils is flagged as one of them, based on their research:

When they look at it, they say "Every time someone eats seed oils, gut permeability increases significantly" - and that allows bacterial endotoxins, LPT, lipopolysaccharides and other things to be absorbed through the gut barrier, and to cause problems in the body. Whether it's autoimmune disease or other problems.

Now, people as they age, we lose some of our digestive capacity. One of the common things we see with people as they get older is their gastric pH goes up. They don't have the capacity to produce a really acidic stomach environment anymore.

Humans have the... are among the most acidic stomach environments on the planet, compared to almost any other animal. We are on par with things like hyenas and vultures - which were scavenger animals! And the thought is:

The reason we developed that is because, initially, when we were an Australopithecine or something like that, we scavenged meat - and that meat was probably sitting out for a while. It was probably heavily contaminated.

So the animals that had a more robust pH that could kill that, outlived the other ones who couldn't. This is the natural selection theory on that.

But as far as: Why somebody would do that? Is a carnivore diet something you can do for a long time?

I mean, I've done it for three years. I had essentially only red meat, with the exception of some fish here and there, some eggs here and there, some spices in case I got to eat in a restaurant.

And three years in, I'm winning World Championships. So if there's an deficiency, maybe it's a ten-year deficiency. I'm kind of skeptical about that.

There's people that have been doing this stuff for 10 years, 20 years, that are still thriving. And it's kind of interesting to see, it just makes sense from an evolutionary plausability standpoint.

If there was some essential plant nutrients, some essential plant food that you had to have to survive... how would you get from Africa to Europe, to Asia, across the Bering Strait, into Alaska, down to North America... what plant would be there that you had to have?

I cannot think of one! If you tell me "*A blueberry is essential for human nutrition*", I'm gonna say "Where did you get blueberries in the Bering Strait, 50,000 years ago, when it's frozen?"

But, it's like: You can always get meat, though!

Bilyeu:
Yeah. Yeah! Look man, so...

One: I love what you're doing with the *N of 1* stuff. I feel like there's a whole movement happening right now, where people are going. "I get it! I don't have proof... but I'm telling you, I'm living it and it's kind of awesome."

Let me back up: So used to be 60 pounds heavier, but not in a good way. All... just fat, a little bit more muscle in fairness.

But mostly, I had putting on muscle when I was on a *SeeFood diet* - so if I saw food, I ate it!

Dr. Baker:
I've been on that one, haha!

Bilyeu:
Yeah. Actually, I was eating so much, I hated eating. It was just "Oh, but I don't want to miss a second to put on muscle!" So I ended up putting on a lot of fat. And I decided "Okay, I'm gonna get lean!" And I did, I got very fucking lean.

And I did it by, basically, rabbit starvation. So I was eating very high protein, probably 80, 85 % of my calories came from protein.

I tried to keep my carbohydrates to zero and I tried to keep my fat to zero. So the 15 percent rest was like stuff sneaking in, just because you can't just eat the chicken breast. But I got as close as I could.

And I did that for two years. I got... shredded would be an exaggeration, but I got very lean. Six-pack abs... and it was miserable! I hated my life! I was hungry around the clock.

My wife and business partners pulled me aside and said "You no longer have a personality!" - and I was like "Wow. I really need to take this seriously!" And the big thing was... I had struggled with this my whole life, I didn't make the connection unfortunately:

My wrists hurt so badly that even in my 20s, I was icing them every night. And I iced them every night for about 15 years! I iced them so much that I had what looked like burn marks on the back of my wrist. That was misery!

Then I met Peter Attia and Dom D'Agostino and they said "Man," this whole keto thing, "you need to be eating fat!" And I just could not wrap my head around that.

I was like "It's called fat, it's gonna make me fat. Like, I'm not gonna eat this stuff!" They're like "Don't be a dumbass, eat it!" So I went into therapeutic ketosis. So I was doing a 4-1 ratio. It was misery, it was gross, I had the keto flu the whole time.

But within three days, my wrist stopped hurting. And I was like "Whoa!!" It is the closest food-related thing to having a drug like effect I've ever experienced in my life!

I went off keto for a year because I had such a bad experience with it. But I kept my fat high and my wrists have never hurt since. That was insanely transformative!

I don't know, 85 like I said 90 percent of my calories now come from red meat and like a nice fatty pork rib. And it's been awesome.

When people started talking about the carnivore diet, I was kind of holding my breath. Like "Am I fucking up my microbiome? Am I moving myself backwards in some way that I can't see yet?" So at one point I pushed hard and I went heavily vegetable.

Because for ethical reasons I would love to never need to eat meat. And I started to feel like shit! Now it's entirely possible I just didn't do it well, I'm willing to accept that. But now, I'm sliding backwards into the most ignorant way of getting in simply red meat - and I feel really awesome!

Dr. Baker:

Yeah! I mean, there's a lot of stuff in there... So I would say, for one:

If we look at, biochemically, what to humans need? What are our essential requirements? There are only essential amino acids, essential fats, vitamins and minerals. That's it. There's no fiber, there's no phytonutrients, there's no other requirements. Those are conditionally. Maybe beneficial, but they're not required.

So if we look at absolute requirements: If you're in rabitt starvation, too much protein... and I would say that, if we look at it evolutionary: I think most humans were getting about 30 to 40% percent of their calories from protein, the majority of the rest would be from fat. And then maybe a few plant foods here and there.

When you go too much on the protein side for too long, that that's a problem. I did something similar, when I went from 300 pounds to 240 pounds in the course of three months, I did the same thing.

I exercised three times a day, I cut my caloric intake in half. I just plowed through it like "I'm just going to do it!" I was at work at a hospital, the nurses said "We liked fat Doctor Baker better because you were not so pissed off and grumpy all the time!"

And it's the same thing, you can't sustain it. You're miserable, you're hungry. This is the thing: For a diet to succeed, you have to...

Well, the two things that make diets not succeed are

1) You're hungry all the time. Because you can't maintain that.

2) The food sucks! Right?

So if you go like "I like eating Oreos and ice cream and Twinkies and cake and cookies. That's good." Now you're gonna say "I can't eat that! But what am I going to replace it with?"

Well, you're gonna replace it with quinoa and kale - and that kind of sucks. But you can say "Hey, maybe if you replace it with steak and eggs..."

Which are - for most people, guys particularly - pretty good stuff, people will say "I can do that. I can replace my old junkfood items with these things." Those are not only satiety producing, they're also very nutritious.

Again, I don't necessarily think everybody needs be a hundred percent carnivore. But when you get your nutritional needs are met through meat - you might add eggs, you might add organ meat (some people are proponents for that) some fish, a little bit of dairy - you are much more likely to be satisfied. You're much more likely to be able to eat infrequently.

When the food is right... I think, the autophagy, intermittent fasting happens naturally. That's what happens. Like, I eat twice a day and that's pretty much my routine. Some days it's once, on occasion it's three times. But it's just, because: I eat enough, I'm satisfied, I eat to my satiety.

Think about it: What other animal needs an app to eat, a micronutrient able to eat, a dietician behind them telling them how to eat? I mean, they just eat! And they don't have chronic disease and they stay healthy!

So there should be a food for humans where you can just eat to satiety, eat when you're hungry - and maintain a healthy level of body weight and avoid disease.

A meat-based diet seems to do that. I say *seems to*, because I'm very biased - I see the results, I see the positive results. Every day, people send me their results.

I'm excited to announce that Harvard's David Ludwig is going to be doing a carnivore study. We're gonna be starting to do that, to get more actual, real modern data on this stuff.

Bilyeu:
Do you know what the study is gonna be? The thing I'm really curious about is: Will it include organ meat? Or are we're just talking like some burgers?

Dr. Baker:
Well, it'll include whatever people are eating. We're gonna try to get as many people in as possible.

Bilyeu:
So this is people already doing it?

Dr. Baker:
Yes, this is people who have already been doing it for six months, it's going to be a survey. It's gonna be looking at their blood work, it's going to be assessing their health.

Obviously, there's a lot of potential confounders and subjective bias, stuff like that. But it's about getting that into the literature. They're going from there and say:

"Look, we have a population of three or four thousand people, that have submitted to us to do a study - and they are either... maybe they're all sick and dying, or maybe they're really healthy." Of which, I think, the latter is going to be the case.

So when we get that into literature, now we have power to say "Okay. Now let's do some intervention trials. Let's see what it does for psoriasis. Let's see what it does for rheumatoid arthritis. Let's see what it does for depression."

Because, anecdotally, I'm just seeing: Every day, I get people writing me "Hey, I had PTSD - it's gone!" Or "It's gotten significantly better."

Bilyeu:
What?!

Dr. Baker:
No, seriously! People say "I had suicidal depression - I don't think about suicide anymore!"

Bilyeu:
Do you think this is inflammation? The less inflammation is bringing that down?

Dr. Baker:
I think it's a combination of things. So if we look at it from a mental health standpoint, we know that creatine, carnosine, carnitine, taurine - all these things are found almost exclusively in meat. Now, granted, your body can make some of that. But when it's at lower levels... and we know that people on plant-based diets have lower levels.

There's a nice study in 2018, looking at carnitine levels: In people with major depressive disorder, their carnitine levels are low. When you supplement carnitine - again, carnitine is a meat based product - their depression gets better. We see that.

So it's probably a combination:

1) Maybe reduction in brain inflammation, but
2) Also supplying these nutrients that have a sort of positive brain chemistry effect.

The thought that nutrition has no role in mental health disease is mind-boggling to me! That people think it does not.

I mean, how could it not? Your brain is just an organ like any other organ in your body, like your liver is. It's subjected to the same environmental goodness and badness that everything else is.

Why wouldn't nutrition have an impact on our brain health?

Bilyeu:
Also, there's a connection from the brain to the gut! In terms of controlling neurochemistry. Huge influence on serotonin, that is almost exclusively stored in the gut, released from there. That one's crazy.

And then, the whole notion of *leaky brain syndrome*...

Dr. Baker:
Right, leaky gut and leaky brain run parallel. If you have a leaky, gut you probably have a leaky blood brain barrier.

Bilyeu:
Yeah. That does seem very striking, that people would push back on that.

One thing I want to know: Like I said, I do sort of a lazy man's carnivore diet. You're the first person I've heard who's actually not pushing organ meat really hard.

You're even saying "Maybe grass-fed is a bit better, but grain-fed's a lot better than going out and eating a Twinkie!"

Do I need to eat the organ meats? Because I really don't want to!

Dr. Baker:
Yeah. It's kind of interesting, I know there's people that disagree with me... and like I said, my whole belief system is *Let me see what the results people are actually having.*

Bilyeu:
The way they feel? Or blood levels? Or something else?

Dr. Baker:
All of it, all of it. Because... the results are generally:

- Are you reversing disease?

- Are you improving body composition?
- Can you subjectively and objectively say you're healthier.

Bilyeu:

But what if you're already healthy? Like, I'm a healthy dude, I'm living a healthy lifestyle since my mid-20s - so I'm not gonna be the guy where you see some massive swing.

I will say from my rabbit starvation: My doctor loved it because my cholesterol was at an extremely low level - but I felt like death. That was not fun!

Dr. Baker:

Yeah, that's a great example of *Great labs - But feel like garbage.*

Bilyeu:

That's what I'm trying to figure out: A guy like me, what should I be paying attention to? Because I've heard you say many times "We're never gonna know if this is gonna make you live longer." Right?

That is an experiment that takes an entire lifetime. So I don't really know - but I want the best guess.

I guess it makes people like sort of giggle under their breath. But, okay: Erections. Like, am I waking up with an erection regularly. I love it, it's a metric.

How do I feel psychologically, a metric. Waist to height ratio, metric. Like, I want to know what are the things, that as doctors get educated:

What should they be looking for, to know whether to assign somebody a carnivore diet - and then, what should they be looking forward to know if the carnivore diet has worked for me?

Dr. Baker:

Right. So I think we have such a sick society right now... there's a study that has come out, saying that 88 percent of us are metabolically unhealthy.

Bilyeu:

Eighty eight?!

Dr. Baker:

Eighty eight percent! There's only 12 percent of Americans that fit a criteria of normal metabolic health parameters. This is why it's just so important!

We have such a disaster... and it's only going to get worse. The problem is with this obesity, diabetic, *diabesity* epidemic, that will turn into a dementia epidemic - and that's impossible to take care of!

When we look at you, the healthy guys. I would say:

Now you're at performance. It's like:

- How fast can I run? How fast getting 100 meters?
- How much can I lift?
- What's my body composition like?
- Am I waking up with a boner every morning?
- Do my joints hurt, does my back hurt?

Those are the things that really matter to you. You could care less what your LDL cholesterol is. If it's 75 and you feel like garbage, it's like "I don't really care about that. I want to feel and perform and do well subjectively, that's part of my life experience." Right?

The thought of *what do we need to eat on a carnivorous diet?* This is the thing: I did a servey a couple months and I got 11,000 responses in 24 hours. And we asked them 25 questions, like "What are you eating?"

The interesting things to me were:

- How many of you were taking prescription medications, and
- How many of you came off of your prescription medications?

And we didn't stratify by period of time, it could have been three months or less. 70% of those people drop their meds!

Bilyeu:
Whoaa!!

Dr. Baker:
So it's like, that is a significant health improvement! Then you say *How many of you guys are eating organ meats on a regular basis?*
Answer: 15 percent. So 85% of the people weren't eating them, either not at all or very rarely.

Bilyeu:
Do you eat organ meat?

Dr. Baker:
I don't, generally. I mean, when it's offered to me... if someone has cooked, I'll eat it. I generally don't like it.

Bilyeu:
Are you eating it because you just like hedging your bets?

Dr. Baker:
No, no. I eat it because I don't know offend the person that cooked it for me. I'm not eating it because I'm worried about some deficiency.
Again: If you look at the people that have been doing this diet the longest, you know, the pioneers... the guys that have been doing it for 20, 25 years: They just eat steaks and ground beef - and they're fine!

Bilyeu:

Alright. Here's a question for you:

Watching a documentary on wolves, the Alpha always gets to eat the... liver, I think it is? Why would that matter if it doesn't have some extra nutrition, some extra value for the animal?

Dr. Baker:

When we look at animals, usually a predator animal is hunting a prey animal that's relatively lean. Thus, protein is not a concern on a meat-based diet. You're gonna get plenty of protein.

What you're not going to get is fat! Where is fat located on a lean animal? It's located in the viscera. So they go after the perinephric fat, the pericardial fat, the omentum. This is where the concentrated fat is. And this is why we see that...

You know, we hear historical accounts of the polar societies where they'll throw the lean meat to the dogs because *I got plenty of protein - what I don't have is fat.*

Remember you, with your sore wrists? All eatin' protein! Like "There's only so much I can eat of that - and then I need some fat!"

So I think it's fat seeking here with the wolves, really. That's why we're cracking bones to get the marrow, that's why we're eating brains because brains are high in fat.

Bilyeu:

Yeah, yeah.

Dr. Baker:

It's not necessarily that there's some magical nutrient in them. And yes, liver has more vitamin E. Yes, the liver has some vitamin C. But I don't think...

Again, I don't have scurvy. I mean, I haven't had Vitamin C in any significant quantity outside of what I get in steaks in three years! With scurvy, Vitamin C is a water-soluble

vitamin. I would just get symptoms within a few months...
and then I would get sick. But we're not seeing that!

Now, some people feel better on that, and I think there are
some people that are particularly vitamin depleted. Them
eating more vitamin containing foods is probably a good
strategy.

You just have to experiment. If you sit there and choke
down a liver, because you don't like it, "I'm just doing out of
my duty." And you say I notice *no improvement*... or maybe
there's some placebo effect where you notice something for
a little bit.

If you don't notice it consistently, maybe you don't need
it.

Bilyeu:
Yeah. agreed.

I can't let you go without talking to you a little bit about
the military. Your experience is all over the map, it's so
fascinating! Like, looking at you, I'm expecting a meathead -
but you're not a meathead! You're a surgeon, you've served
in the military, nuclear launch... officer?

Dr. Baker:
Yeah, I used to be in charge of hundreds of nuclear
warheads, back in the Air Force. I used to be the guy that...
you maybe saw the movie War Games, back in the day.

Bilyeu:
Did you want to be that guy?

Dr. Baker:
You know, it was kind of funny. I went to college,
University of Texas, went to medical school, got roped into
playing rugby. There was this guy, Paul McCartney who was
not from the Beatles... but he had a gym. So he said "You
need to play rugby!" - and so I started playing rugby.

And then I liked rugby and I ended up being pretty good. I got selected on the Western US team, the All Texas Team... then I got recruited to play in New Zealand.

I was like... I'm in medical school and I was like "Hm, fuck it, I'm gonna play rugby in New Zealand!" So I dropped out of medical school, much to the chagrin of my medical school professors. They were like "You you're a good guy, why are you doing this?" I was like "Man, I wanna play rugby!"

So I went there - and then I went into the military as a nuclear weapons officer so I could continue to play rugby, for the military. I played up until I was thirty. And during that time, my day job was nuclear weapons guy. So this was just simply something to do while I played rugby.

And then I got tired of it. I remember, I was playing this team from Russia and I was laying on the bottom of a pile: This guy's kicking me in the head, blood coming out of my ears.

Bilyeu:
Jesus!

Dr. Baker:
I'm like "I'm 30. I'm done, I want to go back!" So I went back to medical school, the military paid for that.

When I got out they immediately... I had to repay my time to them as a surgeon. So they immediately sent me to Afghanistan! And this is like... crazy, crazy time.

Bilyeu:
When was that?

Dr. Baker:
This was 2007. We were in the Afghan war. And it was just... all day long, every day, trauma. Constant trauma. People being blown up, the worst injuries you could possibly see. Little kids, you know. We took care of the Taliban, we

29

took care of the good guys, the bad guys, the civilians... It was just nonstop, it was every single day!

Bilyeu:
How do you deal with that? Like, how do you compartmentalize the trauma? Even just hearing someone scream, I've got to imagine... being back and hearing some someone scream would bring that back. How do you frame that? How do you get over that?

Dr. Baker:
Yeah, it was such a unique situation. Combat trauma, it's just not a normal situation. I mean, the closest thing to that I ever saw as a physician was a refinery explosion, where people were getting blown up. Or a train accident.

But generally, it's so out of the normal realm of my existence, I don't associate anything normal day-to-day with that sort of stuff.

When we were there it was like: All you did was sleep, wake up, eat, operate until you got tired. Try to get some sleep, sometimes operate in the middle of the night - and occasionally exercise. That was it, constantly, every day. And you're just exposed to that.

After a while, you kind of become a little bit immune to it. Because it's like "Oh, another guy's leg's blown off!" - we're used to that.

I remember, when I first got there it was kind of... it was kind of sad. Because I flew in through Kurdistan, we unload our stuff, we're sleeping in this giant hall, like 300 guys on cots. We go in, we hook up with the army. We're the Air Force, we were releaving the army guys.

And in the first night it was "We got to go work!" - we get in there and the first thing I see was this poor dude, he was like a 23 year old Canadian kid:

Both legs blown off above the knee. A Special Ops guy, full beard because they wear full beard in Special Ops. I was just thinking "Holy Shit! Welcome to the war!" This is war in real life... and it just never stopped, from day one. It was just constant, constant trauma.

I don't regret going because I learned a lot. And I was there helping people. I was privileged to be able to help people. But... it's not a good place. It's not. No one should ever look forward to war.

Bilyeu:
Yeah. What did you learn?

Dr. Baker:
Well, I mean, I learned how to improvise, to think fast on my feet. Because when you're as an orthopedic surgeon in the US, you're like "I need this" - and you get all the equipment you need.

But there, you're like "I need a screw that's 44 millimeters long." They're like "We got a 65 and a 20 - so which one do you want?" You don't have the right equipment, the right materials. You're just trying to figure out how to do the best you can with what you have.

It's the unpredictability, a lot of. When I was operating in the US, my goal was to make surgery as boring as possible. Routine. Everything the same way, over and over again. That's what you want.

Over there, it was like... you don't know what you're gonna get. You don't know if you're gonna have the equipment. We ran out of saline... there's no water! We were doing surgery, we don't any have saline to rinse wounds or wash our hands? I mean, what are we gonna do? You just don't have a choice.

So sometimes you learn that you can do a lot more than you think you can.

Bilyeu:
That's really just incredible! Like, I can't imagine how that begins to shape the way that you think. Did it change the way that you think about people, about humanity, about your job?

Dr. Baker:

I think it made me not fear things. Because now I'm like "Anything that someone throws at me, I've seen much worse!" Particularly from a medical standpoint. It's kind of like *I've seen the worst of the worst that you can possibly imagine.*

As I do what I'm doing now, I get a lot of negativity thrown my way - and I'm like "Pff! What am I worried about?" So I just kind of laugh at that stuff.

It made me a harder person, a tougher person. Not a mean person. I still care very much about people. But at the same time, I'm kind of imbued with this resilience to keep forging ahead, despite what seems to be a lot of opposition.

What I'm doing obviously is controversial, with regard to diet. There's a lot of pushback, there's a lot of status quo that does not want to be disrupted.

There are a lot of people that are happy to provide you with pills for your various ailments and illnesses, and manage your disease. And that's a billion, trillion dollar industry.

We're all thankful that there's medications that may help us in a certain situation. But we would much rather not have them in the first place.

Bilyeu:

Yes, very much so. Which leads me to my last question. But before I ask that: Where can people find you online?

Dr. Baker:

I am active on social media, Instagram. I'm on Twitter, I have got a YouTube channel *Shawn Baker MD.*

This is important: We're starting a company called **MeatRX.com** - it's going to be a giant resource for people that are interested in learning more about diet, all the scientific references that support this.

We're gonna have some coaching component, for people that want to have some support as they do this. That's something I'm pretty excited about.

Then, of course, my book is coming out: *The Carnivore Diet* by Shawn Baker. Knock on wood that it does well!

Bilyeu:
Nice man, that's exciting!

So to the end, that we would much rather just not get sick than have something to treat it: What is one change that people could make that would have the biggest impact on their health?

Dr. Baker:
Yeah. I think ownership, taking ownership of your own health is probably the biggest thing people can do. Because too many people outsource their health to other people!

I'll speak from the perspective as a physician: Yeah, I want to help you. But I don't have as much invested in your health as you do! So you have to take ownership of your own health. And you have to be willing to see what actually works for you.

So I think we have to step outside the box and say "What is actually helping me?" Be objective about it, measure what's important to you. Not what's important to somebody else! Measure what's important to you.

Because ultimately, you've got to live in that space. You've got to live in that body. And if your labs look great but you feel like garbage, there's something still wrong. So you have to be willing to be your own guide for some of this stuff.

Bilyeu:
Right, I love that! I couldn't agree with that advice more.

Take things into your own hands - you should be doing an experiment on yourself, you should be figuring out what works for you.

It's always interesting when people are so even keel, to have clearly a strong belief about how things should be - but can also say that

"Hey, at the end of the day, it's gonna be up to you. Try it, see if it works for you. If it does, great. If it doesn't, move on and try something else!"

Until next time my friends: Be legendary and take care!

Chapter 2
Nutrition, Exercise, and Healthcare

How many of you guys have heard about the carnivore diet? I want to see your hands up. Hands up everybody! So, pretty much everybody in the room. That's good, okay.

How many of you guys - since hearing about it - have either adopted a carnivore diet or started adding more meat into your diet? That's, again, a lot of the people in the room.

So of you guys that have adopted a carnivore diet or added more meat into your diet, how many people have noticed a benefit in their health or their physical performance? So many? Wow! Again, so... that's all we need to say really guys! I mean, meat's good food.

The important point I want to make is: As you guys are probably painfully and acutely aware, there is a very well funded, very well organized and a very aggressive campaign globally to get you and I to stop eating meat.

They want us to stop eating meat to save the environment, to save our health... and they are putting it in messages in schools, teaching little kids that meat is bad. This is something that we as a community have got to step up and say "Enough is enough!"

Because I will tell you: The beef industry is not going to do it. I've talked with the beef industry and 80% of the beef industry is controlled by three major companies. They're going to be selling plant-based burgers too, guys. So it's up to us to make a change. I just wanted to get that out of the way and try to motivate some people to step up.

All right, let's talk a little bit about *nutritional heresy*, the carnivore diet. Maybe it's not so heretical at all - but just for the sake of talking about why it might be beneficial.

So when you first hear about the carnivore diet, most people say, like I did: "What the heck are you talking about?!" Right? That's the normal response and I don't blame people for that response. But as we go on, we kind of say "Well, what is a carnivore?"

What's a Carnivore

- An animal that eats meat
- Obligate Carnivore
- Falcutative Carnivore
- HyperCarnivore (70%)
- Omnivore
- Herbivore

- Every Nutrient we need to thrive is contained within another animal

The simplest definition if you look in the dictionary, it's an animal that eats meat. Humans eat meat, so we're carnivores. Now, there's different categories in there:

There are obligate carnivores. These are animals that absolutely must eat meat to survive. This would be like a cat. There's something called a facultative carnivore which I think human beings are - and that means they do better when they include a significant part of meat in their diet.

There are hyper carnivores which is defined as when about 70% of your diet comes from meat. Omnivores, obviously. they eat meat. And surprisingly, even animals classified as herbivores, will eat meat when they get the chance.

They're just not very good hunters. Cows are not great hunters. But if they can catch a little chicken or a little bunny running around, they'll eat it!

Think about it: We are made up of fats, proteins, vitamins and minerals. And everything that we need as a human to survive is contained within another animal - that's just the bottom line there.

Are humans just a bunch of meat-eating savages? This is a picture of the Lascaux paintings in France.

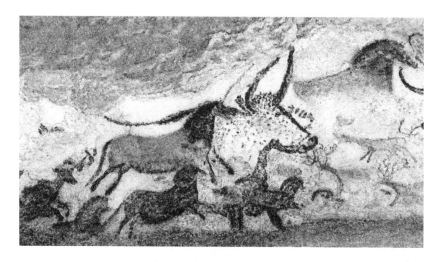

These are famous cave paintings from about 40,000 years ago. If you go there, you cannot actually see these paintings. They've actually reproduced it in a cave next door because they're so precious. This, to me was a menu, guys! This is one of the early menus, that was a restaurant.

These are some savage people that still do this today, eating a raw caribou carcass. Humans do this.

When we look at some of the stable radio isotope data that's come out from the Max Planck Institute and other scientific places, we see that:

When we look at the collagen of fossil Remains, it clearly shows that humans ate as much meat or more meat than other carnivorous animals like wolves.

Stable radioisotope data repeatedly shows high level carnivory in both Neanderthal and Homo Sapiens

Isotopic evidence for the diets of European Neanderthals and early modern humans

Michael P. Richards[a,b,1] and Erik Trinkaus[c]

[a]Department of Human Evolution, Max Planck Institute for Evolutionary Anthropology, Deutscher Platz 6, D-04103 Leipzig, Germany; [b]Department of Anthropology, University of British Columbia, Vancouver, British Columbia V6T 1Z1, Canada; and [c]Department of Anthropology, Washington University, St. Louis, MO 63130

Edited by Richard G. Klein, Stanford University, Stanford, CA, and approved June 23, 2009 (received for review April 7, 2009)

We report here on the direct isotopic evidence for Neanderthal and early modern human diets in Europe. Isotopic methods indicate the sources of dietary protein over many years of life, and show that Neanderthals had a similar diet through time (~120,000 to ~37,000 cal BP) and in different regions of Europe. The isotopic evidence indicates that in all cases Neanderthals were top-level carnivores and obtained all, or most, of their dietary protein from large herbivores. In contrast, early modern humans (~40,000 to ~27,000 cal BP) exhibited a wider range of isotopic values, and a number of individuals had evidence for the consumption of aquatic (marine and freshwater) resources. This pattern includes Oase 1, the oldest directly dated modern human in Europe (~40,000 cal BP) with the highest nitrogen isotope value of all of the humans studied, likely because of freshwater fish consumption. As Oase 1 was close in time to the last Neanderthals, these data may indicate a significant dietary shift associated with the changing population dynamics of modern human emergence in Europe.

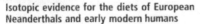

Exceptionally high δ15N values in collagen single amino acids confirm Neandertals as high-trophic level carnivores

Klervia Jaouen, Michael P. Richards, Adeline Le Cabec, Frido Welker, William Rendu, Jean-Jacques Hublin, Marie Soressi, and Sahra Talamo

PNAS March 12, 2019 116 (11) 4928-4933; first published February 19, 2019 https://doi.org/10.1073/pnas.1814087116

Edited by Richard G. Klein, Stanford University, Stanford, CA, and approved December 21, 2018 (received for review August 16, 2018)

Article | Figures & SI | Info & Metrics | PDF

Significance

Identifying past hominin diets is a key to understanding adaptation and biological evolution. Bone collagen isotope studies have added much to the discussion of Neandertal subsistence strategies, providing direct measures of diet. Neandertals consistently show very elevated nitrogen isotope values. These values have been seen as the signature of a top-level carnivore diet, but this interpretation was recently challenged by a number of additional theories. We here apply compound-specific isotope analysis of carbon and nitrogen in bone collagen single amino acids of two Neandertals. These Neandertals had the highest nitrogen isotope ratios of bulk collagen measured so far, and our study confirms that these values can be most parsimoniously explained by a carnivorous diet.

Slide 1

That was what our history indicated. That is a pretty big clue, and the science on this is really, really solid.

If we look at one of our early predecessors, Homo Erectus: Human beings have been on earth roughly about three million years. If you believe in evolution - I realize there's people out there that have a creationist view.

Food of choice from Homo Erectus onwards was megafauna, particularly probscideans

Elephant and Mammoth Hunting during the Paleolithic: A Review of the Relevant Archaeological, Ethnographic and Ethno-Historical Records

Abstract

Proboscideans and humans have shared habitats across the Old and New Worlds for hundreds of thousands of years. Proboscideans were included in the human diet starting from the Lower Paleolithic period and until the final stages of the Pleistocene. However, the question of how prehistoric people acquired proboscideans remains unresolved. Moreover, the effect of proboscidean hunting on the eventual extinction of these mega-herbivores was never seriously evaluated, probably because of the lack of acquaintance with the plethora of information available regarding proboscidean hunting by humans. The aim of this paper is to bridge this gap and bring to light the data available in order to estimate the extent and procedures of elephant and mammoth hunting by humans during the Quaternary. This study examines the archaeological evidence of proboscidean hunting during Paleolithic times, and provides a review of ethnographic and ethno-historical accounts, demonstrating a wide range of traditional elephant-hunting strategies. We also discuss the rituals accompanying elephant hunting among contemporary hunter-gatherers, further stressing the importance of elephants among hunter-gatherers. Based on the gathered data, we suggest that early humans possessed the necessary abilities to actively and regularly hunt proboscideans; and performed this unique and challenging task at will.

Slide 2

But if we think about evolution, Homo Erectus kind of figured out how to hunt. These were the guys that kind of did it for us. So about a million and a half years ago, they became very effective at hunting something called probsidians, which are mammoth mastodons and elephants. And that was what they selected for, because these animals don't run away.

When think about it: If you see an elephant in the wild and a lion comes up to it, it doesn't run away. I've been to Africa and seen herds of elephants. And when you look at them, you stop in front of them - all they do is turn and face you... and say "What are you gonna do?" Because you're so little.

But Homo Erectus figured out that these elephants wouldn't run, so they're just a big giant blob of calories. You just got to get a spear in them and they're gone, and they were very efficient at hunting them.

This paper basically says *human beings could kill mammoths at will* - so anytime they wanted. That's an important thing to know.

Africans have been hunting elephants forever.

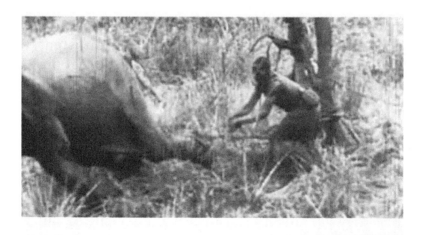

Native Africans hunting elephant 1930s

One of the reasons we think that elephants still predominate in Africa and not in North America, like there used to be and not throughout Europe, is: When humans

39

evolved in Africa, elephants kind of knew we were there and so they were a little more wary.

But once we migrated out to Europe and then Asia and then across the Bering Strait to North America, South America, those animals didn't see what was coming! So we were able to just decimate them.

This is another thing, the evolution of our stomach acids and its relevance to our human microbiome.

RESEARCH ARTICLE

The Evolution of Stomach Acidity and Its Relevance to the Human Microbiome

DeAnna E. Beasley 🔘, Amanda M. Koltz, Joanna E. Lambert, Noah Fierer, Rob R. Dunn

Published: July 29, 2015 • https://doi.org/10.1371/journal.pone.0134116

Slide 3

If we look at the list inside this study, when we look at the gastric pH of human beings, we are almot on top of the list! Our gastric pH is about 1.5. It's very important to note that most herbivores, their gastric pH is about 4, 5, 6 - some of the carnivores have a gastric pH of about 2 or 3.

And then humans uniquely, among a few other animals, have a gastric pH of about 1.5 - that is consistent with vultures, hyenas and other scavenger animals. That probably gives us clues, again, how we evolved. We evolved probably scavenging behind big cat predators.

There's some studies out of Africa showing that a lion will typically leave about 20 kilos of meat behind, from a zebra kill. And so the humans probably went up there, after the lion was done ... or they scared them away if they were brave enough. We still see Africans doing this today!

Then they got this meat, but it had been sitting out for a while. It probably had some contamination - and that's why they evolved the gastric pH of 1.5. Now, the other theory behind that... there is interestingly another animal that has a low gastric pH, that's an herbivore - it's called a rabbit.

40

The reason rabbits have low gastric pH is because they eat their own poop. So we could either say humans ate meat or they ate their own poop - I think the more likely explanation is that we ate meat.

All right. This is a study Felisa Smith did out of the University of New Mexico.

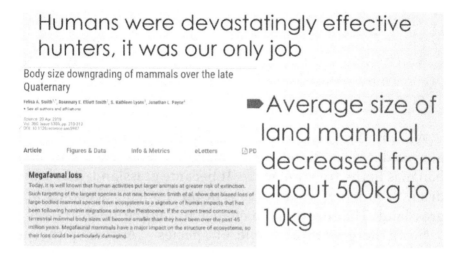

Humans were devastatingly effective hunters, it was our only job

Body size downgrading of mammals over the late Quaternary

➡ Average size of land mammal decreased from about 500kg to 10kg

This is really interesting: At the beginning of the pleistocene - which occurred about 120,000 years ago... if we took all animals, cats, dogs, rats, rabbits, elephants, camels and we averaged their size 120,000 years ago, the average size of an animal was 500 kilograms!

If we look at that today, in North America, it's about 7.9 kilograms and worldwide, it's about 10 kilograms. And so all of that meat, all of that yummy tasty fatty meat, just disappeared. Now, some people say it's climate change, most of the paleo zoologists will say *probably overhunting by man*. Probably a combination of the two depending on the area. But: We lost most of our food.

Temperature: So if we look back about three million years ago, on this top graph we see what happens.

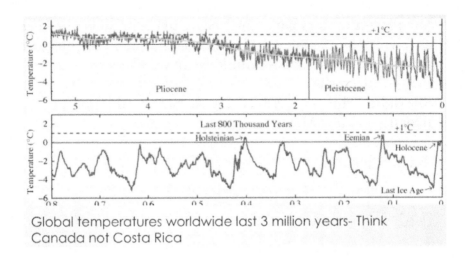

Global temperatures worldwide last 3 million years- Think
Canada not Costa Rica

We were in a very warm period and then it got cold. As it got colder, we didn't have mangoes and coconuts and bananas in the trees anymore. It became grassland, it became drier. So much of what humans or pre-humans occupied was grassland. That drove us to change our nutritional strategy.

Now, there were a couple of species - Australopithecus Robustus and Australopithecus Boisei - that tried to go the vegetarian route. They went extinct. Right? So that kind of tells us something there.

They already did the vegan experiment for us and they went extinct, so we don't need to continue playing with that.

And then, this is the last 800,000 years on the lower graph, and it shows you: Generally, the temperatures were very cold. And if we look at the farthest edge of the graph, where we are today, we are in an extremely warm period! Okay?

So think about Canada, rather than Costa Rica - this is kind of the environment that humans evolved in!

This is an interesting study, done a couple years ago.

Human weaning times are predictive for carnivory based on brain mass

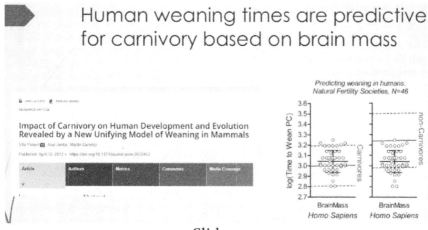

Impact of Carnivory on Human Development and Evolution Revealed by a New Unifying Model of Weaning in Mammals

Ella Pelland, Axel Janke, Martin Garwicz

Published: April 18, 2012 • https://doi.org/10.1371/journal.pone.00.02452

Predicting weaning in humans:
Natural Fertility Societies, N=46

Slide 5

So if we look at all animals, all mammals - mammals are defined because they breastfeed - if we look at their brain growth and their brain mass relative to weaning time, and what kind of food they choose...

We know that human beings have the largest brain of any primate for sure. We have the shortest weaning time of any primate! And so the only way that humans could reasonably grow a brain the size of it is, is by including extremely energy high, calorically rich foods. Primarily carnivore food which include animal fat. That's extremely important.

On average, wild humans will breastfeed about two and a half years, looking at indigenous tribes. We don't do that so much, in modern society it's usually six months to a year, some people do it longer. Now we have high calorie, sweetened, fake Formula... high calorie sugary food which makes up for some of that energy deficit. But that's not what we're designed for!

If we look at any other animal this would predict humans are carnivorous.

This is another nice study that Miki Ben-Dor and others did.

RESEARCH ARTICLE

Man the Fat Hunter: The Demise of *Homo erectus* and the Emergence of a New Hominin Lineage in the Middle Pleistocene (ca. 400 kyr) Levant

Miki Ben-Dor, Avi Gopher, Israel Hershkovitz, Ran Barkai 📧

Published: December 9, 2011 • https://doi.org/10.1371/journal.pone.0028689

Article	Authors	Metrics	Comments	Media Coverage

Early man preferentially sought out fat for fuel

Slide 6

So when you're eating animals, it's easy to get protein. Protein is not a problem. And we had these giant elephants and mammoths, so that's what man preferentially sought. They sought out fat. What happened is:

When the fatty animal supply went away... a mammoth or an elephant is usually about 60 percent fat by volume, you look at a nice source of fat meat...

When that ran out, we had to adopt a different strategy. So what happened? Again, we lost all those animals, I talked about how the animals got smaller. Then, we had to develop agriculture to meet our nutritional needs. I mean, we just ran out of energy, there was an energy crisis! So we developed agriculture.

It allowed us to have civilization, that was good. I mean, it saved the species, right? Because there's no more food left. It allowed the species to flourish and to have more people. But what happened to the human being?

Dawn of agriculture took toll on health

Date   June 18, 2011

Source   Emory University

Summary   When populations around the globe started turning to agriculture around 10,000 years ago, regardless of their locations and type of crops, a similar trend occurred: the height and health of the people declined. The pattern holds up across standardized studies of whole skeletons in populations, say researchers in the first comprehensive, global review of the literature regarding stature and health during the agriculture transition

1

Brain size decreased by about 200cc

Stature decreased by around 6 inches

Muscle and skeletal density decreased

Dentition became poor

Slide 7

If we look back 100,000 years ago compared to what happened after farming occurred, our brain size actually shrunk by 200cc! So we had a smaller brain.

We shrunk about six inches. Our muscle density and our skeletal density got weaker - and our teeth turned awful! We got smaller jaws... we just became a less robust species, when we adopted a plant-based, grain-based agricultural diet.

All Right. So the carnivore diet: I wrote a book called *The Carnivore Diet* so I have the liberty to kind of define this. This is how I like to define it:

Carnivore Diet- What is it?

➡ A dietary strategy that focuses on utilizing nutritionally dense animal based foods that either limits or eliminates plants as needed with the goal of improving health

It's not about ethics. It's not about saving the environment. It's not about *saving the broccoli or the carrots*. **It's about doing what works for you and focusing on what you need.**

45

That doesn't mean you've got to eat nothing but meat and salt and water! Some people need to do that, for sure. Some people feel better with that. But find where your level is - and many people find that less plants, more meat, is the key. Okay? So that's how I define this.

So, for anybody trying to make their definition - that's how I define it. What does the carnivore diet not do?

It won't regrow limbs, okay. You won't fly or have other superpowers... although being healthy today might be a superpower, quite honestly. And you won't live forever! Well, I don't know... so far I haven't died yet. Maybe I will, we'll have to see.

This is the thing: A lot of people criticize and say: Well, it only works because... and then we'll talk about: What are those *becauses?*

It only works because...........

- It eliminates junk food/irritants
- It doesn't irritate the gut
- It mimics fasting
- It reduces food cravings
- It's simple
- It's nutrient dense
- It's high protein

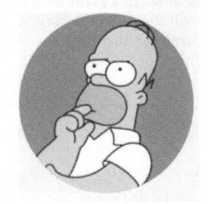

It eliminates junk food. Right? It eliminates garbage from your diet. Well, okay! Great, you're not eating garbage, that's a good thing!

It doesn't irritate the gut, which is true. So people say "Well, that's one of the reasons it works."

The carnivore diet works because it 'mimics fasting'...so maybe we should just not eat at all! Not only not eat meat, just don't eat it all.

It reduces food cravings, so you're not drawn to the cupcakes or the pizzas or all those foods. I mean, they taste delicious! There's no doubt about it.

It's simple... it's even lazy. Why would you do something that's not complicated? Why would you do something that doesn't require 10 apps and a fitness tracker, macronutrient balancing and micronutrient balancing - why would you do that?

That's silly, it doesn't make sense. Humans shouldn't do that, we need complexity to eat.

It's nutrient dense and it's high in protein. I mean, there's more protein than the average diet. Now, you may have a fatter version but you're getting a lot more protein.

So when I look at that, I say "All those criticisms of why it works, I'm seeing that overall, it's a pretty damn good diet if you ask me!"

Some of the criticisms out there.

Criticisms

- Lacks phytonutrients
- Potential vitamin or mineral deficiencies (vit c...)
- Devoid of fiber
- Its not balanced
- Brain needs carbohydrates to function
- Protein stimulates mTOR and leads to aging and cancer
- Meat is bad for us (obesity, heart disease, cancer, diabetes)
- Meat eaters are bad people (vegans)

There's no phytonutrients... these valuable, wonderful phytonutrients that no human being had ever heard of, prior to a hundred years ago. That we had no idea we're supposed to eat them.

We probably had no clue what sulforaphane was. I mean, those things are so valuable we have to eat them. Broccoli, which wasn't introduced into the american diet since 1920 is something we have to eat now?

So potential vitamins and mineral deficiencies. I'll talk a little bit more about that, Vitamin C being the major one that's often cited.

There's no essential fiber. *You've got to have fiber or your colon is going to fall out! You've got to have fiber or these bacteria in your microbiome are going to revolt and start eating you from the inside out!*

It's not 'balanced'... I'll put one ribeye in my left hand and one ribeye in my right hand, that's a balanced diet for me!

But... you know, "It's not balanced!" - and no one defines *balanced!* What is a balanced diet? I don't know, *eat a bunch of colored stuff, get as many as you can and that's going to be balanced.*

Your brain has to have carbohydrates to function. *If you don't get 130 grams of carbohydrates, you'll to stop thinking!* And some people argue that's happened to me and I'm brain dead, so on and so forth. But I would beg to differ.

This is the latest hot topic, protein: "Oh my god, protein stimulates mTor - and you're going to die and get cancer if you eat any protein!" So we've got to not eat protein. We've got to eat the bare minimum amount, right?

Meat is bad for us, it makes us fat. Gives us heart disease, cancer, diabetes. We hear that all the time. And then just: *Meat eaters are just bad people in general!* This is something the vegans will tell us, "You're just a bad person if you eat meat!"

All right, let's talk about a little bit about this: Phytonutrients.

Phytonutrients- Zero essential requirements, generally poorly absorbed, positive effects generally seen via upregulation of endogenous detoxification systems

Comprehensive REVIEWS In Food Science and Food Safety

Comprehensive Reviews in Food Science and Food Safety   Free Access

The Role of Dietary Phenolic Compounds in Protein Digestion and Processing Technologies to Improve Their Antinutritive Properties

Tanja D. Cirkovic Velickovic, Dragana J. Stanic-Vucinic

First published: 28 November 2017 | https://doi.org/10.1111/1541-4337.12320 | Cited by: 7

Digestion is the key step for delivering nutrients and bioactive substances to the body. The way different food components interact with each other and with digestive enzymes can modify the digestion process and affect human health. Understanding how food components interact during digestion is essential for the rational design of functional food products. Plant polyphenols have gained much attention for the bioactive roles they play in the human body. However, their strong beneficial effects on human health have also been associated with a negative impact on the digestion process. Due to the generally low absorption of phenolic compounds after food intake, most of the consumed polyphenols remain in the gastrointestinal tract, where they can exert inhibitory effects on enzymes involved in the degradation of saccharides, lipids, and proteins. While the inhibitory effects of phenolics on the digestion of energy-rich food components (saccharides and lipids) may be regarded as beneficial, primarily in weight control diets, their inhibitory effects on the digestion of proteins are not desirable for the reason of reduced utilization of amino acids. The effect of polyphenols on protein digestion is reviewed in this article, with an emphasis on food processing methods to improve the antinutritive properties of polyphenols.

Slide 8

There is zero essential requirement for phytonutrients in the human diet. There are none that we require!

Think about it: Let's say that there's some magical phytonutrient in a blueberry and you're going to say "Well, that blueberry didn't grow in Alaska in January, where would I get that magical required phytonutrient?" There is nothing...

I would challenge anybody to name one plant that you can't live without - and there's the answer is going to be *none!* We can look at some of these things. Phytonutrients sort of cause a hormetic effect and some attribute benefits to them.

They say "Well, it toughens you up! It stimulates the NRF pathways, it simulates the cytochrome p450 system. It upregulates that, therefore you're more robust and you can handle other insults." There are other ways to do that:

Exercise will do that... hell, breathing pollution will actually do that! Not that I'm advocating sucking on a tailpipe - but if that's your argument for eating plants, we have to realize there are negative effects of these same 'wanted' compounds.

We talk about polyphenols, *they're great! Everybody's got to eat polyphenols!* Well, polyphenols interfere with the absorption of amino acids - things you actually need! And so it's kind of like "Okay, maybe it's going to upregulate your liver detoxification system - but at the expense of not allowing you to absorb essential nutrient requirements!" So there's a good and a bad. I think you have to figure out where you fall on that.

Phytonutrients are less bioavailable. In my view, as an athlete, the only beneficial role I see to plants is a readily available supply of glucose. And that may or may not be helpful for certain people. But I don't see that there's any reason to eat plants outside of glucose, quite honestly. I know that's a controversial statement.

So RDAs, nutrient deficiencies, let's look at the evolution of the RDAs.

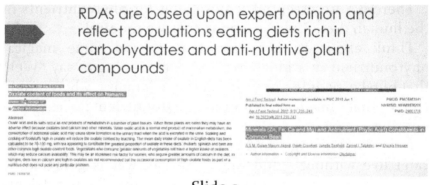

Slide 9

So in 2007, the Institute of Medicine reviewed the RDAs, and their conclusion was: *The RDAs are based on expert opinion.* This is the lowest level of evidence that we have! Okay? So our entire nutritional science is found on some guy pulling it out of his butt, saying "This is what everybody's supposed to eat."

I mean, we're supposed to get the RDA for everything. But realize, the RDA was based on a grain eating population, eating things that interfere with the absorption. We know clearly that fiber will inhibit absorption of various minerals, things like iron, calcium, magnesium and zinc.

We know that phytic acid does the same thing. We know oxalates will do the same thing. So if we're eating a diet rich in that stuff, guess what? Our nutrition requirements go up!

When we take that stuff out of the diet, it changes completely our nutritional requirements. That's one thing to think about.

Some Vitamin C stuff, just because everybody's worried about scurvy: I've been doing this diet for nearly three years now. There are people who have been doing this diet for over 20 years. I've seen literally thousands upon thousands of people doing a carnivore diet - I've seen exactly zero cases of scurvy! Right?

We would think "Well, maybe somebody should get scurvy by now" - no one has gotten scurvy. Now, if you want to get scurvy, eat a crappy junk food diet with no fresh food at all, and eat beef jerky. Then you'll get scurvy. But no one's doing that, no one's recommending that.

So we know, just for the sake of completeness, Vitamin C is competitively inhibited by glucose. That is to say: If there's a lot of glucose around, the transporters which transport Vitamin C into the cell - whether it's across mitochondrial membranes and across the gut membranes - is competed. Therefore, you absorb and can utilize less Vitamin C.

Vitamin C actually can be recycled by the red blood cells, humans have the capacity to recycle used Vitamin C, which is very interesting. One of the functions of Vitamin C is that they are antioxidants. We always hear about the antioxidant property of Vitamin C.

Well, we know when we go on low carbohydrate diets - and the carnivore diet is a low carbohydrate diet for sure - we see an upregulation of our natural antioxidants. Things like glutathione and other things are elevated so the Vitamin C antioxidant property is less required.

It's also involved in carnitine production. Carnitine is something that helps with fat metabolism - and if you look at the root of the word *carn-* or *carnivore*, carnitine is found heavily, heavily in meat. Particularly red meat.

I think it's found... like asparagus is like the only vegetable you might be able to find it in. But generally, you're going to see an increase in carnitine consumption. And then the other thing, about collagen...

Interestingly, 20 years ago, we used to think that the only way you can absorb amino acids were individual amino acids. So phenylalanine, tyrosine, tryptophan, all those things would be broken down and we'd absorb them through transporters. But they've discovered that in the gut, there are di- and tripeptide transporters - therefore you can you can absorb these molecules like carnosine, like carnitine.

And when it comes to collagen: Hydroxyllysine and hydroxyproline, which Vitamin C converts to - it converts proline and lysine to hydroxylproline and hydroxyllysine... so when you have that absorbed directly: If you're eating collagen or collagen precursors, it goes directly in! That's helpful for collagen production.

The problems with scurvy are: Your teeth fall out, your joints hurt, your skin is easily hurt because the collagen production is compromised. And we've known for 140 years, that fresh meat will prevent scurvy. That is well known, there's no question about that.

Let's talk a little bit about fiber. We're told that fiber is essential, there's all these benefits to fiber and... I don't disagree with that! I think fiber can be potentially beneficial - and again, I think it is conditional.

Fiber

- Non- essential, but conditionally somewhat beneficial in context of omnivorous diet
- Satiety
- Glucose mitigation
- Minimally positive effects on weight loss, blood pressure and cholesterol
- The microbiome (SFA Butyrate)

Let's talk about that. So it's not essential but conditionally, somewhat beneficial in a context of an omnivorous diet. It does or can have a satiety effect, right? You can fill yourself up with indigestible material and you'll get full. You could eat rocks, you could eat cardboard - you could accomplish the same thing with regard to that.

It may mitigate glucose response, so if you swig a big glass of apple juice and then put your glucose monitor on, you'll see a big spike. If you do that compared to an apple, you'll see less of a spike, so it may mitigate that.

And we do know that preventing huge swings in glucose is very important, particularly those big highs above 140 milligrams per deciliter. But guess what? When you're on a carnivore diet guess what happens your glucose? Flat line! So it's not even an issue.

You know, the randomized controlled trials and interventional trials on fiber show minimal to no effect on weight loss, blood pressure and cholesterol. And again, the whole thing about cholesterol: Many of you guys in here are sophisticated enough to know that cholesterol may or may not be an issue, depending what else is going on.

Then, the microbiome: This is a new topic, this is the latest thing that the cerial manufacturers are telling you, right? This is where this stuff comes from, quite honestly. "Eat fiber to protect your microbiome! You gotta develop those short chain fatty acids. It's so important! If you don't have it, your colon is gonna stop working and you're gonna die!"

No Fiber

- Satiety generally improved on a meat based diet
- Lack of high glycemic foods on carnivore diet renders glucose mitigation benefit moot
- Carnivore diet generally results in weight loss and normalized blood pressure, cholesterol is a no longer a black and white issue
- Microbiome science is still in its infancy but butyrate can be easily supplied to colonocytes by the reversible reaction of the ketone body BetaHydroxyButyrate that is up regulated via a carnivore diet

So without fiber... again, most people that are going on a meat-based diet notice an incredible sense of satiety. I say *most people* - some people don't, but most people do. That kind of negates the satiety effect.

Again, the lack of glycemic high glycemic foods: With a carnivore diet, most people note weight loss is better. Most people note their blood pressure gets better, probably due to vascular inflammation going down.

Cholesterol... again, not a black and white issue, in my mind at least. And the microbiome science: Remember, we're still naming microorganisms that live in the gut. We don't even know what's in there, yet.

There's studies out there that show that the stool samples you send off to you Ubiome, it doesn't even match what's actually going on in the colon. There's studies out there to show if you send three stool samples, they'll all be different! So we really don't know that much about the microbiome.

But the thing about butyrate... yeah, we know that short-chain fatty acids are elicited by the fermentation of fiber by bacteria. Butyrate - now, most of you guys know about ketones and ketosis, and some of you guys have heard of betahydroxybutyrate, right?

Betahydroxybutyrate is basically just an OH-molecule attached to butyrate! That is a reversible reaction, that happens very easily. So if you are making ketones - and you do on a carnivore diet or a low carb diet - those ketones also get to the colonic epithelial cells, which this butyrate is supposed to be helping. And guess what: It quickly interchanges and you have the same protective effects. So you don't need fiber to get butyrate.

This is a study that was done, I think 2012, Anne Peery did this.

Gastroenterology. Author manuscript: available in PMC 2013 Jul 26   PMCID: PMC37

Published in final edited form as: NIHMSID: NIHMS3

Gastroenterology. 2012 Feb; 142(2): 266–72 e1   PMID: 22(

Published online 2011 Nov 4. doi: 10.1053/j.gastro.2011.10.035

A High-Fiber Diet Does Not Protect Against Asymptomatic Diverticulo

Anne F. Peery, Patrick R. Barrett, Doyun Park, Albert J. Rogers, Joseph A. Galanko, Christop prevale and Robert S. Sandler   divertic

Slide 10

It was a colonoscopy study, looking at a couple thousand people. Where they actually looked at what was going on inside their colon. They looked at it and they found the people with the highest amount of fiber, the people that had the most bowel movements, had the greatest amount of diverticulosis.

Diverticulosis is a little outpouching that occurs... it's like a little balloon that pops out of your colon, and then stuff like seeds and other crap gets stuck in there, then it gets inflamed and you get a diverticulitis. Then you get put on antibiotics or you get your colon whopped out.

So diverticulosis occurs in people that eat *more* fiber! And it went down: The lower fiber you ate, the less you had. Okay?

Another study was done out of Korea. It showed that people that had constipation, chronic constipation... the only way they got rid of it was to go no fiber at all! People had ate more fiber, their constipation got worse. Their bowel movements became less frequent.

World J Gastroenterol. 2012 Sep 7; 18(33): 4593-4596.
Published online 2012 Sep 7. doi: 10.3748/wjg.v18.i33.4593

PMCID: PMC3436786
PMID: 22969234

Stopping or reducing dietary fiber intake reduces constipation and its associated symptoms

Kok-Sun Ho, Charmaine Yeu Mei Tan, Muhd Ashik Mohd Daud, and Francis Seow-Choen

▸ Author information ▸ Article notes ▸ Copyright and License information Disclaimer

RESULTS: The median age of the patients (16 male, 47 female) was 47 years (range, 20-80 years). At 6 mo, 41 patients remained on a no fiber diet, 16 on a reduced fiber diet, and 6 resumed their high fiber diet for religious or personal reasons. Patients who stopped or reduced dietary fiber had significant improvement in their symptoms while those who continued on a high fiber diet had no change. Of those who stopped fiber completely, the bowel frequency increased from one motion in 3.75 d (± 1.59 d) to one motion in 1.0 d (± 0.0 d) (P < 0.001); those with reduced fiber intake had increased bowel frequency from a mean of one motion per 4.19 d (± 2.09 d) to one motion per 1.9 d (± 1.21 d) on a reduced fiber diet (P < 0.001); those who remained on a high fiber diet continued to have a mean of one motion per 6.83 d (± 1.03 d) before and after consultation. For no fiber, reduced fiber and high fiber groups, respectively, symptoms of bloating were present in 0%, 31.3% and 100% (P < 0.001) and straining to pass stools occurred in 0%, 43.8% and 100% (P < 0.001).

Slide 11

So basically, you've got a traffic jam and you're just shoving more cars in there? I mean, that's not the way you do it, you kind of have to get rid of the cars.

There's a polyp prevention trial.

Cancer Epidemiol Biomarkers Prev. 2007 Sep;16(9):1745-52.

The polyp prevention trial continued follow-up study: no effect of a low-fat, high-fiber, high-fruit, and -vegetable diet on adenoma recurrence eight years after randomization.

Lanza E[1], Yu B, Murphy G, Albert PS, Caan B, Marshall JR, Lance P, Paskett ED, Weissfeld J, Slattery M, Burt R, Iber F, Shike M, Kikendall JW, Brewer BK, Schatzkin A; Polyp Prevention Trial Study Group.

Slide 12

So they were looking at people that had adenomas, cancerous lesions or pre-cancerous lesions in their colon. And they looked at fiber - and adding fiber and fruits and vegetables to that did nothing to help it. Nothing whatsoever! There's a lot of literature out there that supports that fiber is kind of overrated.

All right, a balanced diet. Again what does it mean? I think it's because you're eating the wrong food! You're eating a nutritionally inferior food. Because you've got to cobble together as much as you possibly can to try to make it nutritionally complete - when you should have just eating a big old hunk of steak and you'll be fine.

Another argument: The brain needs carbs! Right? I've already gone over this stuff, I'm not dead yet. The brain needs glucose, right. We know we need some amount of glucose and there are other cells in our body that need some glucose. I mean, red blood cells, renal medulla, some of the testicular cells...

Our brain needs glucose to some degree. Although Cahill back in the 1960s with his starvation studies showed: People with the blood glucose down around 10 or 20 milligrams per deciliter were fine! As long as they had adequate ketone production. So how much we need is debatable.

You clearly will make glucose. The nice thing about being on a low carb or carnivorous diet is: You will make the glucose you need, it's very much a demand-driven process for the most part. So that's a very nice way to regulate your glucose, based on need, not based on erratic supply.

Because when your supply is erratic, it just goes up and down, up and down, up and down.

Okay, mTor.

mTOR

- Almost entirely from low level animal studies on flies, worms and mice, no credible human data

- Insulin and overconsumption of food is a much more potent stimulator of mTOR

This is a really interesting topic that I've kind of delved into quite a bit. I don't have a lot of slides on this... but:

Most of the evidence on mTor shows that if we limit protein in lower level animals, like fruit flies, like worms, rats and some of these other animals, that they tend to live longer. Same thing with caloric restriction.

Well, I'm not a fruit fly, I'm not a worm or a mouse - there is really no credible data whatsoever in human populations.

Walter longo and crew had done a study based on epidemiology. But if you listen to criticisms from guys like Don Layman and some of these other protein researchers... it was absolutely just abysmal what they did with the data!

So there's no credible human data that shows that reducing protein is going to help you in any regard for living longer or for not getting cancer. In fact, we see what happens to people that restrict their protein.

The American population: If we go to any nursing home, we see nothing but frail, sickly, old elderly people. And I cannot tell you how many old people whose broken hips I've taken care of - and they are underprotein for sure!

Insulin, the overconsumption of calories - if we're worried about mTor - is the biggest driver of mTor! So if you're eating eight times a day, eating your carbohydrate-based snack every 3 hours, you're going to be spiking mTor all day long!

Whereas, what happens to most people on a low carbo-hydrate diet, or carnivorous diet, is: They eat very discreetly, they eat a couple meals a day. Once, twice a day, sometimes three times a day. They have a very short protein spike and they have very little chronic mTor stimulation.

Also, we're finding out that mTor is differentially stimulated in different tissues. That is to say: Sometimes if I eat protein and exercise, mTor is going to be spiked in my muscle where I need it, I want to have lean muscle. But it doesn't occur in other tissues where you might have a problem. So we realize, it's more nuanced.

This is the thing, anytime we discover some new thing, whether it's the microbiome, whether it's mTor - we all get excited... or insulin. We all get excited "Oh my gosh, the answer is zero! I gotta make it all zero!" That's not good, the body is more nuanced and more complex than that.

We have to keep that in mind, that mTor is needed. There's a reason we have it. Cholesterol is needed, there's a reason we have it. Insulin is needed, we there's a reason we have it.

Meat equals cancer, diabetes, heart disease, early death

- Almost completely based on unreliable epidemiology studies of low relative risk that do not satisfy basic Bradford Hill criteria for causation and are wildly confounded by healthy user bias, short term trial looking at often nebulous biomarkers and on animal or in vitro studies that cannot be extrapolated to humans
- No Randomized controlled trials demonstrate these conclusions

- Should we accept poor science as a basis to make population wide recommendations because it's too hard or too expensive to do good science?

I mean, literally, there is no credible information that would suggest that. There's a lot of epidemiologic studies out there. I'm sure you guys are aware of the healthy user bias:

You'll take 50,000 people, you'll hand them a food frequency study, ask them what they ate the last six months. They guess, they don't know. You put the people in there, they're smokers, drinkers, overweight, the diabetics... the people that just don't care.

You put them in one group and you compare them against the people that exercises, people that don't drink, that wear their seat belt, that eat fruits and vegetables and fiber - because they're told it's good for them, and they're generally healthy. And they exercise. Of course, there's a difference!

But there's no good data on that stuff. Epidemiology is largely just garbage. We need to stop doing that. This is Harvard Harvard School of Public Health, putting this stuff out continuously.

The risk numbers are so low... I mean, the relative risk numbers are low. The absolute risk numbers are extremely low. There's no randomized control trials to demonstrate these conclusions.

This is why you have to find out this information. And there probably never will be, there will never be a 75-year randomized control trial using twins, locked in a metabolic ward, controlling every variable and altering their diet. That's never going to happen.

So for these people that think that you can use these studies to tell you what you or I need to eat to be healthy 50 years from now... it's literally witchcraft! It's religion, it's astrology. It's just silliness.

Should we accept this poor science to make population-wide recommendations for every single person to eat? And I think the answer to that is clearly no.

All right, again: Meat eaters are evil. Right?

Meat Eaters Are Evil

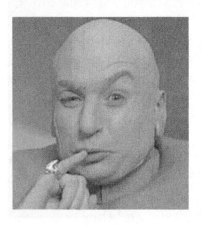

➡ Long topic but the entire Paleo/low carb/keto/carnivore community needs to stand up to this garbage

This is what we hear: "You're ruining the planet. You don't care about it. You're mean to animals. If you eat a steak, it's equivalent to going and kicking a chicken in the head," that's what they think you're doing.

I mean, it's a long topic. But again, this is something that I think we need to push back on hard. If you look at the people that actually raise animals - and there are exceptions out there - these people spend their lives learning how to take care of animals, and they care about them!

And I think we as a community of meat-eaters, it's on us to make sure that industry is done appropriately. It's not that we don't care about animals, but we realize: We need to eat them and they're part of our nutrition and part of our health.

What are we seeing with people that go on a carnivore diet?

What we are seeing

- Resolution of metabolic disorders -not surprising given the data we already have on low carbohydrate diets
- Improvements in HDL, Trig, Insulin sensitivity, Inflammatory markers, blood pressure, body composition, NAFLD, Autoimmune disease, IBS and IBD, Mood, depression, Anxiety, Skin Disorders and musculoskeletal problems (arthritis, tendinitis) and quite a bit more

A lot of metabolic disorders are going away. What we know about low carbohydrate diet is already in the science, it's not surprising at all.

We generally see an improvement in things like HDL, triglycerides, insulin sensitivity, inflammatory markers, blood pressure, body composition, non-alcoholic fatty liver disease... autoimmune diseases, which is very fascinating!

Irritable bowel syndrome, inflammatory bowel disease, mood, depression, anxiety, skin disorders, muscle skeletal problems. Arthritis, tendinitis - and quite a bit more. So it almost sounds like a panacea! I just think good nutrition...

I don't think there's a single chronic disease out there - including cancer - that does not get affected by nutrition, good quality nutrition. If anybody asked me "What do you think about this weird crazy disease?" I've never heard of, my standard answer is "Good nutrition is likely to help!"

We just have to realize that. And it surprised me how much it does help. And it's not all down to weight loss. A lot of people will say "Well, it's just because they lost weight." I've seen skinny people that had autoimmune diseases, that were underweight, get better. Because they improved their nutrition quality. So it's not all just down to weight loss.

I've seen people with severe *I need a knee replacement-joint pain...* I'll put them on a ketogenic or a carnivore diet, their pain will go away. Without losing any significant weight. It's more than just the weight loss.

All right, what are some of the potential mechanisms?

Potential mechanisms

- Improved nutrition quality and bioavailability
- Decreased stimulation of chronic insulin over secretion
- Restoration of compromised intestinal permeability (leaky gut syndrome)
- Removal of potential toxins/problematic foods (seed oils, sweeteners, refined grains, phytotoxins)

Again, better nutritional quality. I'll stand up here all day and say *meat is better nutrition than plant food*. It just clearly is. It's better in bioavailability, there's over stimulation of insulin. Like I said, you got to stimulate some insulin, but less overstimulation.

Likely, it helps with restoring intestinal permeability, the so-called leaky gut. There's pretty good evidence out there that shows that leaky gut tends to contribute to a lot of these things - and removing potential irritants seems to help significantly.

Then again, removal of problematic foods. I mean, seed oils, sweeteners, refined grains, phytotoxins. Those things for me are a no-brainer, but it's kind of controversial.

These are some people that have been doing it for a while.

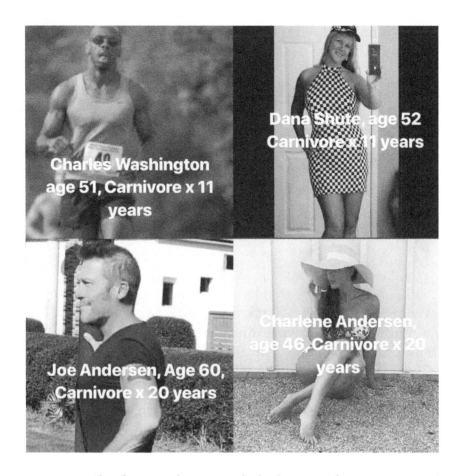

Charles Washington age 51, Carnivore x 11 years

Dana Shute, age 52 Carnivore x 11 years

Joe Andersen, Age 60, Carnivore x 20 years

Charlene Andersen, age 46, Carnivore x 20 years

We got Charles Washington, he's doing it for 11 years. He's a marathon runner in his 50s. Dana Shutes, 52 years old, been doing it 10 years. Joe and Charlene Anderson... I mean, Joe is 60 years old, on the bottom. Charlene is 46 - they've been doing carnivore diet for 20 years. None of them have scurvy! Or at least, if they do have it, they look pretty good for scurvy patients.

And then world-class athletes, - I've got world-class athletes right now that are doing it.

World class Athletes

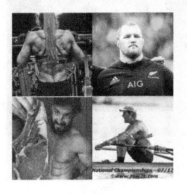

- Sarah Thakray- BJJ World Champ
- Owen Franks- New Zealand All Blacks Rugby
- Paul Jordan- Larochelle French Professional Rugby
- Michael Clouhger- US Men's National rowing team

We've got Sarah Thackray, who's a world Jiu Jitsu champion on a carnivore diet for a year. We've got Owen Franks, New Zealand All Black rugby player. The New Zealand All Blacks are the most successful athletic team of all time of any sport! He's one of the best rugby players in the world, on a carnivore diet for now almost two years.

We got Paul Jordan, another professional rugby player in the French league. We got Mike Clouhger, who is on the US national rowing team. He's the fastest rower on the team - and he's on a carnivore diet! So athletes performing on this.

I've got an olympic shot putter that I'm consulting with. Also, he likely will meddle in the Olympics as a carnivore. So pretty amazing.

So controversies in the carnivore diet. Do we need to eat organ meats? Do we need to eat eyeballs and brains and livers... and eat it all raw? Stuff like that?

Controversies

- Necessity of Organ meats
- Collagen supplementation (methionine/glycine ratios)
- Ideal fat/protein ratio
- Cooked vs raw/rare
- Long term deficiencies
- Seasonal variations in diet (berries in the summer/fall)
- Suitability for all

Again, I'm gonna say that this is controversial. Do we need to supplement collagen? Do we need to be sprinkling collagen powder on our steaks to balance the methionine-glycine ratio?

What is the ideal fat to protein ratio? I think there's a lot of controversy in there because some people find... myself in particular, when I want to get really lean, I eat leaner, I eat more protein. There's other people that doesn't work for. And I think it really depends on your particular metabolic situation, your goal and athletic desires.

That's controversial: Do we need to cook the meat or should we eat it raw? Should we eat it like those those people in Northern Russia, should we all just be eating raw meat?

Are there long-term deficiencies? Again, maybe there will be. I haven't seen it yet, but maybe there will be. And then, seasonal variations. Humans obviously walked by a patch of berries and ate some. I would! I'd eat Twinkies if they were available 50,000 years ago. I mean, you would eat whatever's available.

Is there a benefit to that? Maybe, maybe not. It depends on the person, I'm kind of open-minded about that. And then, is it suitable for all people? The answer for me is: I think all humans can eat meat. Does everybody need to, want to... would they do better on a carnivore diet? I certainly don't know the answer to that. I think it's something to experiment with.

All right, where do we go from here?

Where do we go from here

- ➡ Most of data is anecdotal (Stefansson Bellvue studies 1928, PaleoMedicina Group)
- ➡ Physicians adding case repots to literature
- ➡ Intervention trials
- ➡ Support for sustainability practices (Joel Salatin, Gabe Brown, Alan Savory)

We have a lot of anecdotal data. We've got a couple of literature studies, we've got Vilmar Stefansson's studies from 1928 when he came back and sat in a lab for a year, and he ate all meat - and lo and behold, nothing bad happened to him. He was fine. That was back in 1928, though, and there were six peer-reviewed studies that came out of that.

The Paleomedicina group in Hungary has got a number of case reports, doing basically a meat-based diet, which is showing reversal of Crohn's Disease, reversal of ulcerative colitis, reversal of type 1 diabetes if you catch it early enough. So all these interesting things.

I would like to see if there's some healthcare providers and physicians out here, let's start getting some case reports in the literature. I talked with the National Cattlemen's Beef Association and their research team about how do we get research funded - and they're kind of on the fence right now. Because they're kind of tied up by the USDA and they won't let you say too much.

But once we start getting case reports in the literature, it'll open up some more research, with intervention trials.

Like I pointed out at the beginning: We need to support sustainable agriculture, guys like Joel Salatin and Gabe

Brown, Alan Savory, so on and so forth. That needs to be a bigger part of our agriculture production systems. It doesn't have to completely replace that - but I think we need to really show that that can be effective, and support those people. For those that have the ability to do that. Okay, I think that's all I have.

So any questions?

Question:

I'm wondering, at what point in your carnivore like journey can you start cutting out supplements? Or are there certain supplements that you would recommend to keep. Because I still take probiotics, magnesium, iodine, things like that.

Answer:

Yeah. I can't give you a blanket answer on that... I don't take any supplement. I mean, I take salt if you consider that a supplement. I use Redmond Real Salt.

It's going to depend on where you came from, why you're taking it. I think from an athletic standpoint, a lot of people do feel electrolyte support does seem to help them. Those other things: What I would do is just eliminate it for a while and see how you do.

Here's the thing with me: When I went on an all meat diet, it was like "Wow! This is a big difference!" I noticed things. When I take a supplement... I've been lifting weights, doing athletics stuff, I would take supplements, I'd buy the chromium pecanalate and the latest products. And you'd be like "Meh, I can't tell if it helped!"

If you get this *I can't tell if it's helped,* then why are you paying money for it? That's how I would approach that, just see what happens to you. Because at the end of the day, it's all about

- how you function
- how you feel
- how you look
- how you perform
- how your systems are working.

And if the supplements aren't really clinically doing something for you, I'd really question why you'd be taking them. Okay? Hopefully that helps.

Question:
Hi Dr. Shawn, I just wonder what your take is on fast food burger patties, like what your favorite is? For me, Burger King... because they're bigger.

Answer:
This is controversial because I go... once in a while, while I'm driving and I'm hungry... this is the thing:

Fast food companies generally suck. They put out garbage. They've made so many people sick with their cokes and their fries - fried in seed oils - and their frosties and all that stuff. It's not good food.

However, most places have 100% real beef. Most people think it's filled with crap, and some places do have crappy fillers and stuff like that. But most places don't. So if you're on the road or on the go and you want to do that as a quick easy meal, I'd say that's fine.

In fact, we have fast food places in every small town in America. We could literally solve much of our obesity and diabetes problems by just telling people "Go in there and eat burger patties!" Because the distribution system's already set, right? I talk about this in the book a little bit.

While I think it's important to support regenerative agriculture and sustainable agriculture, I still think meat is good, regardless. Not to plug them, but I go to Wendy's a lot, just because I like the way they taste. They use a little more fat in their burgers, I think they taste better.

It's always like this, I do it kind of sneakily. Because I'll ask them "Hey, do you guys sell single burger patties?" before I even order. Then they got to find it in their registry, and they got to bring the manager up to figure out how to bring it up.

So they bring it up and they say "Oh yeah, it's right here. It's a $1.29." I say "Okay, great! Give me 12 of them!" - and that's how I get it done! I don't mess around with *I want a burger without a bun*.

At the beginning of the deal, I'd negotiate the price and whether they have it - and then I order. So that's how you got to do it.

Thank you guys!

Study Sources Chapter 2

[The Slides with numbers in the Text do include scientific sources]

Slide 1

Michael P Richards, Erik Trinkaus:
Out of Africa: modern human origins special feature: isotopic evidence for the diets of European Neanderthals and early modern humans
Proc Natl Acad Sci USA, 2009.

Klervia Jaouen et al.
Exceptionally high δ 15 N values in collagen single amino acids confirm Neandertals as high-trophic level carnivores
Proc Natl Acad Sci USA, 2019.

Slide 2

Agam Aviad, Barkai Ran:
Elephant and Mammoth Hunting during the Paleolithic: A Review of the Relevant Archaeological, Ethnographic and Ethno-Historical Records
Quaternary, 2018.

Slide 3

DeAnna E Beasley et al.
The Evolution of Stomach Acidity and Its Relevance to the Human Microbiome
PLoS One, 2015.

Slide 4

Felisa A Smith et al.
Body size downgrading of mammals over the late Quaternary
Science, 2018.

Slide 5

Elia Psouni, Axel Janke, Martin Garwicz
Impact of Carnivory on Human Development and Evolution Revealed
by a New Unifying Model of Weaning in Mammals
PLoS One, 2012.

Slide 6

Miki Ben-Dor et al.
Man the Fat Hunter: The Demise of Homo erectus and the Emergence
of a New Hominin Lineage in the Middle Pleistocene (ca. 400 kyr)
Levant
PLoS One, 2011.

Slide 7

Emory University
Dawn of agriculture took toll on health
2011
https://www.sciencedaily.com/releases/2011/06/110615094514.htm

Slide 8

Tanja D Cirkovic Velickovic, Dragana J Stanic-Vucinic:
The Role of Dietary Phenolic Compounds in Protein Digestion and
Processing Technologies to Improve Their Antinutritive Properties
Compr Rev Food Sci Food Saf, 2018.

Slide 9

S C Noonan, G P Savage
Oxalate content of foods and its effect on humans
Asia Pac J Clin Nutr, 1999.

ASM Akond et el.
Minerals (Zn, Fe, Ca and Mg) and Antinutrient (Phytic Acid)
Constituents in Common Bean
Am J Food Technol, 2011.

Slide 10

Anne F Peery et al.
A High-Fiber Diet Does Not Protect Against Asymptomatic
Diverticulosis
Gastroenterology, 2012.

Slide 11

Kok-Sun Ho et al.
Stopping or reducing dietary fiber intake reduces constipation and its
associated symptoms
World J Gastroenterol, 2012.

Slide 12

Elaine Lanza et al.
The polyp prevention trial continued follow-up study: no effect of a low-
fat, high-fiber, high-fruit, and -vegetable diet on adenoma recurrence
eight years after randomization
Cancer Epidemiol Biomarkers Prev, 2007.

Chapter 3
Tailoring the carnivore diet for specific goals

Host Vinnie Torturich:

You know who this guy is and if you don't, get over to Instagram right away! I was shocked to see him with a shirt on - usually he doesn't have one on. He's working out topless most of the time... but if I'd look like that, I wouldn't even own a shirt.

He's been on our show before, he's got his own show. You need to go check this guy out, he's got a lot of stuff going on online.

Look, I don't invite very many people over. But he's that kind of guy you just want to invite over again. I'm talking about Dr. Shawn Baker!

Shawn, welcome to the show. I'm going to leave it to you now.

Dr. Shawn Baker:

Hey Vinnie, thank you so much for having me. It's an honor to be with you guys, with all your audience. With all that great people that you had before and will have after me. So this is a real privilege.

I'm going to talk about a little bit different stuff today. Well, it's still obviously stuff we're learning about the carnivore diet. But I'm not going to try to convince people *why you should do a carnivore diet* or what the rationale in it is.

But it's more what we've kind of learned over the last couple o fyears as we get more and more data. I'm gonna share my screen now and just get into this, and then I'll try to leave room for questions.

THE CARNIVORE DIET

LESSONS FROM THE FIELD

Okay, so the title of this talk is "The Carnivore diet - Lessons from the Field". So this is just some of the stuff we've learned over the last several years, as I've been both a very vocal advocate of the carnivore diet, and learning from research from other sources. Then, of course, the experiences of the community and myself.

I do have some conflicts of interest:

DECLARATIONS

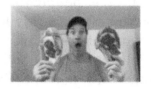

- Author of book "The Carnivore Diet"
- CEO of MeatRx.com
- Dedicated Meat Eater

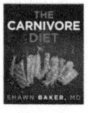

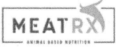

I'm the author of a book called *The Carnivore Diet.* I'm the CEO of a company called *MeatRX.com* which is a large community platform that is dedicated to helping people improve their health, using animal-based nutrition.

And I am certainly a dedicated meat eater! So take everything I say with a grain of salt because I am certainly conflicted... although I try to be truthful as much as possible. That's my intention, to be truthful based on what I know.

Okay, so where's the information I'm gonna share with you coming from?

WHERE IS INFO COMING FROM

- Historic
    - 1928 clinical trial (2 people x 1 year, Steffanson, Andersen)
    - A few isolated case reports (eg PaleoMedicina, Clemens, Toth)
    - Historical population observations

- Studies in process
    - Harvard, Lennerz, Ludwig- 2,000 subject observational study (6 months)
    - RCT Carnivore diet funding/design

    - Continuously daily feedback from 4,000 member group at MeatRx.com hundreds of consultations

There's some historic stuff: Obviously, most people are aware that there was a large year-long clinical trial back in 1928.

Two people, one was a guy named Vilhjalmur Steffanson and Carsen Andersen, were put in a metabolic ward for a period of time. They were followed for a year, eating an all-meat diet. As they had claims that they they had done so successfully, after spending up to a dozen years in the arctic with some of the inuit populations.

The main nutritionists of the day didn't believe it was possible. Basically, out of that experiment, I think six highly appreciated studies came out... or popularized peer-reviewed studies were generated from that particular experience.

We've got some isolated case reports. And in more recent literature, a group out of Hungary - led by Doctors Csaba Toth and Zsofia Clemons from the Paleomedicina - published a number of articles on carnivore diets.

There are obviously historical population observations we can kind of draw some of our conclusions upon.

There are currently some studies in process, which is a new development. Belinda Renerts and David Ludwig, Belinda is a primary investigator, David is a senior investigator, they are looking at information from 2000 people that have been on a carnivore diet for at least six months, doing an observational study.

That is ongoing, the data collection period is over. Basically, the datasets are getting written up and are hopefully ready for publication later this year.

And then we're trying to get a randomized control trial, an intervention trial going - which is currently in the funding and design stages. Thankfully, we just launched that a week ago, we've already raised something like 53,000 dollars for that, trying to get to 200,000 dollars.

Then, I spend every single day, seven days a week, basically since we launched MeatRX - without a day off - I spend an hour with our community. And we constantly get feedback. We're constantly checking what is going on in the community, what people are trying. What things are people finding out.

And we're starting to get some data that's converging on what things are working for what people, and how to kind of tailor this diet based upon who you are and what your situation is.

This is something that is important. There's not a *just go do one thing approach* and it works for everybody. So we're learning as we go.

So what is the carnivore diet, for those who don't know that?

WHAT IS THE CARNIVORE DIET

- Non Dogmatic, not "reverse Veganism"
- Do what works best for you not your ideology
- Some people include a modest amount of plants in their "Carnivore diet"

- "A nutritional strategy that focuses on obtaining nutrients from animal sources and either significantly limits or fully eliminates plant foods AS NEEDED to obtain improved health or performance"

Well, first of all, I'm not very dogmatic about this. Although there are people within the community that tend to do that. But: It is not reverse veganism, okay? At least, I am very much an advocate of doing what works best for you - and not your ideology! Okay?

Some people include a modest amounts of plants in their carnivore diet... goodness gracious, isn't that a controversial statement. This is all about what is working best *for you.*

As someone who kind of wrote the book *The Carnivore Diet, popularized* the name - I didn't invent the name carnivore - but I think I was the first one to attach that phrase with this style of eating. So I've taken some liberty on how I define that.

The way I like to define it is:

A nutritional strategy that focuses on obtaining nutrients from animal sources - and either significantly limits or fully eliminates plant foods **AS NEEDED** (I put the as needed in bold there because that's a critical phrase) - *to obtain improved health and performance or performance.*

We're looking at what works for you to reach health goals. We're not out there trying to save the tomatoes, or save the cucumbers, or save the broccoli. This isn't a religious ideology. All we're looking at is human health - and that is the overarching goal for why we do what we do.

I know it goes against what a lot of people believe, what a lot of the nutritional dogma shows - but at the end of the day, we are results based.

Okay. Why does it work?

WHY IT WORKS

- "It's all about hormones/calories"
- YES, you can get fat or sick eating zero carbohydrates, however it is hard and most do not!
- Wrong amounts of the wrong foods (Dairy, fat, protein)

- Satiety
- Protein
- Elimination of garbage (NSNG, seed oils etc....)
- Simple
- Non inflammatory
- Restoration of gut health

People may say "It's all about hormones" or "It's all about calories in, calories out." Well, quite honestly, none of those statements are true. There's contributions from both of those. Yes, you can get fat or sick, eating zero carbohydrates. Believe it or not. However, it is difficult for many, and most do not.

Why would people get fat or sick? Because they're eating, quite honestly, the wrong amounts of the wrong foods. And those can be fat, protein... and sometimes dairy can be an issue for people.

Why does it seem to work? For one: Satiety. If you don't overeat because you're satiated, that is very helpful. Then: The high amounts of protein. This tends to be, but not always... and I'll talk about different situations where this is true.

It tends to be a higher protein diet than the typical american diet. The typical american diet ranges from about 12 to 16% of its calories coming from protein. Many, if not most people on a carnivore diet, are eating 20, 30 even 40% of their calories coming from protein.

So protein does seem to have some unique metabolic effects. Whether it's the thermic effect of protein, whether it induces greater NEAT (Non-Exercise Activity Thermo-genesis), there are some unique aspects of protein.

The elimination of garbage food and *no sugar no grain,* that our host Vinnie is so fond of talking about. The seed oils, etc. Clearly, we're getting rid of junk food. It's hard to do a junk food meat diet. So that is a big effect.

It can be simple... or it is simple. For a lot of people it is as simple as *Hey, go eat a bunch of meat 'till your full and you're done.* That helps with compliance.

When you're constantly having to calculate macronutrients, when you're constantly having to weigh your food, that gets frustrating over time. Many people have a difficult time adhering to that. So simplicity seems to be another thing.

It is non-inflammatory - despite what you might hear from the plant-based camps. What we are seeing consistently is this tends to be an extremely non-inflammatory diet.

As we have come to learn, that gut health is vital, it has a vital role in in our overall health - and this diet also seems to be very, very effective at restoring gut health.

All right, some variations:

VARIATIONS

- Strict Carnivore
  - IBD (Crohn's, Ulcerative colitis, +/- IBS)
  - Severe Autoimmune issues
  - Refractory Mental Health Disorders
  - Severe food addiction

  - Ruminant meat, salt, water, +/- organ, relatively high fat (75% or higher)

So which people would benefit from a more strict version of a carnivore diet? Like I said, there's different degrees of people that adhere to, various strictness. Now, people that are dealing with IBD (Inflammatory Bowel Disease), Crohn's disease, ulcerative colitis disease. I put +/- IBS in there, IBS is not truly considered an inflammatory bowel disease - but many people with IBS do benefit from going fairly strict.

People with severe autoimmune disease. People with refractory mental health disorders, whether it's bipolar, major depressive disorder, anxiety... we've even seen things like post traumatic stress disorder improve.

People that are dealing with severe food addictions, and there are many people that deal with that. People that have binge eating disorder issues.

What does that look like? It's usually some type of ruminant meat - and when I talk about ruminant, I think Peter Ballerstedt either already talked or will talk to you about that. You will probably learn what a ruminant is:

That's an animal with a multi-chambered stomach. Cows, goats, sheep, and a lot of the wild game would fall into that category.

So ruminant meat, salt. Saltwater plus or minus organ meats. And this often tends to be in a relatively higher fat situation, 75% or even higher.

VARIATIONS

- Relaxed Carnivore
  - Obesity
  - DM
  - Metabolic syndrome
  - Osteoarthritis
  - Metabolically healthy
  - Athletes

  - Red meat, seafood, shellfish, pork, poultry, wild game, eggs, organs, +/- Dairy, seasonings, spices, variable fat content (50-80%)

There's a sort of a more relaxed carnivore diet, I'll describe what that is below. But people dealing with this kind of run-of-the-mill, plain old obesity, diabetes, whether type 1 or type 2, metabolic syndrome, osteoarthritis as opposed to inflammatory arthritis, like rheumatoid and psoriatic arthritis.

People that are otherwise metabolically healthy. And then generally athletes. This is: Red meat, seafood, shellfish, pork poultry, wild game, eggs, organs, plus or minus dairy.

Again, dairy can be problematic for some people. Seasoning, spices... and the fat content for this tends to be variable. Fifty percent, eighty percent, depending on what your goals are.

Diabetes. This is a this is an interesting topic:

DIABETES

- Support of HCP is essential (they may not agree, but will need to assist with med adjustments)
- Cautions with sulfonylureas, insulin as incidence of hypoglycemia is very possible
- Rarely DKA reported with SGLT2 inhibitors and ketogenic diets
- Glycemic control appears to be better on a higher fat (75-90%) approach, to include fat fasts
- Sources of fat, beef fat, suet, bone marrow, brain, pork belly, egg yolks, sausage, less desirable are dairy fats, butter, ghee, cream
- Protein is lower and titrated to glycemia, protein tolerance can improve with time
- Limit Hepatic GNG precursors rather than glucose uptake by muscle etc (GLUT4)
- Fasting +/-, Exercise
- Overeating equals weight gain and poor outcomes

One thing I'll say if you're a diabetic: The support of your healthcare provider is essential! When you're going on a carnivore diet, or really any low-carb diet. They may not agree with your dietary choice but they still are going to need to assist you with medication adjustments.

Most diabetics that go on low carb diets - including carnivore diets - will need to adjust their medications. I should also put that hypertension is another one, and there are a few other medications out there. So if you are on multiple medications, it's probably a good idea to consult with a health care provider.

If your physician is opposed to it, it might be time to get a new physician. We maintain a huge list of physicians that are low carb friendly over at Meatrx.com, if you're looking for one. But regardless, a healthcare provider is is helpful. Sulfonylureas... diabetics probably know what these are, caution with sulfonylureas and insulin.

As the incidence of hypoglycemia is very possible. particularly early on, hypoglycemia can be a deadly complication. And so it's it's not something to ignore. You have to be very cognizant of the fact, you need to be able to figure out how to correct hypoglycemia.

It's usually some sort of dietary intervention that raises blood sugar quickly. Whether it's a carbohydrate source, it's typically utilized for that. So a lot of people use orange juice or glucose tablets or something like that. That's something to realize when you first get on the diet.

I believe that there's been some rare cases of DKA, diabetic ketoacidosis associated with SGLT2 inhibitors. With ketogenic diets, I haven't seen that with a carnivore diet yet. But a carnivore diet certainly can be a ketogenic diet. So if you're on those medications, that might be an issue, although it's pretty rare, pretty uncommon.

Again, glycemic control appears to be better on the higher fat approach to the carnivore diet. To include a *fat fast*... and in fact, we just had a discussion with this with our group this morning. A lot of people are doing that.

Basically, what is a fat fast? That means you only eat fat for a day. That is something that people are seeing extremely, extremely tightly controlled glycemic levels with, with very low blood glucose numbers. We're seeing diabetics that typically run 120s, 130s, 140s, that are seeing numbers in the 70s and 80s pretty reliably with that approach.

That's something that is emerging as a strategy within that. And there's some literature on very low calorie ketogenic diets, showing similar stuff in the literature - which would be consistent with that.

Sources of fat that people utilize, beef fat: You can literally go to your butcher, your supermarket, and ask the butcher to save the fat trimmings for you. It often helps if you call ahead. They're more than happy to do it because they just throw it away anyway. And so people are finding that by taking that, they'll often give you four, five, six pounds of it.

You just cut it up into pieces, you can throw it in the pan, fry it up with some salt, throw it in the air fryer. It is incredibly delicious, it's amazing that they throw this stuff away! If you like bacon, you'll love this stuff. I mean, it's got that really just fat, salty taste which wonderful.

Suet, which is also fat around the internal organs, typically the kidneys. Bone marrow, brain, for people that like to eat that. Pork belly, egg yolks. Certain sausage is high fat, you want to avoid the stuff that has the garbage in there.

And less desirable, quite honestly, are the dairy fats: Butter, ghee, cream. Some people can work those in. But generally, I recommend staying more towards the actual true animal fats and not the dairy fats.

Protein intake is typically lower for diabetics, and we titrate it to glycemia. So what you want to do is: You titrate up your protein based on your blood sugar. And protein tolerance does seem to improve over time as these diabetics get metabolically healthier.

There's some evidence in the literature... actually, there's quite a bit of evidence in the literature that the beta cells can improve over time. We see that the beta cells, what happens to them:

Some of them differentiate, some of them stop losing insulin secretory capacity. But they're still there! So type 2 diabetics, in many cases 60% or more of their beta cells are still active.

Even type 1 diabetics have a small amount of living beta cells. So some question is: Maybe there might be a little bit of recovery there. That's very controversial, but I have seen a number of type 1 diabetics that now are on the minimal dose of insulin - and even a few of them that have actually come off insulin! Which, I know, is shocking and controversial. But it is what it is.

Now, there's some concern - Ben Bickman and I had this discussion the other day - about the fact that he's seeing that as well. And it may be that they're misclassified. Maybe they're really MODY, which is maturity onset diabetes in youth. And that is why we're seeing these type 1 diabetics come off of their insulin completely. So that seems to be a very interesting experience.

And again, we often talk about insulin resistance. In fact, the muscles cannot take up glucose because the insulin-mediated glucose transporter is being inhibited by different compounds, ceramides and things like that.

There is some evidence that hepatic gluconeogenesis is maybe the primary driver of hyperglycemia, rather than the insulin resistance. That is to say skeletal muscles can still uptake glucose, despite the insulin resistance.

Fasting seems to be very helpful for some of these people. Some people need to do it, some don't.

All right. So a carnivore diet for the metabolically healthy and for athletes:

METABOLICALLY HEALTHY/ ATHLETES

- Higher protein approach (fat 50-80%)
- +/- minimum effective dose of well tolerated carbohydrate sources
- Protein 1.2-2.2+ gm pro/kg bodyweight (ballpark estimate)
- May rely on dairy if tolerated for weight gain if desired
- Muscle gain
  - Protein goals
  - Meal frequency increased up to Q3-4 HRS (mTOR stimulation via leucine 2.5-3gm)
  - Post work out protein (carbohydrate unnecessary) 1-2 hrs post workout
  - CALORIC SURPLUS (may require eating past satiety)

The higher protein approach is often utilized. Fat can be 50 to 80% of the diet at maintenance. Some folks will be able to use some carbohydrates. When I'm dealing with athletes and they want to use carbohydrates, we try to figure out what the minimum effective dose of well tolerated carbohydrate sources is.

When I say *well tolerated,* it's GI tolerability: Does it lead to issues with recovery, inflammation? Those things. Protein in these cases tends to be higher than the RDA, 1.2 to 2.2 grams or more per kilo of body weight is a ballpark estimate.

I don't get too prescriptive about this. But in general you have to see what works there.

Some will will tolerate dairy and rely on that. Dairy can be a source of nutrition, particularly when weight gain is desired, it has a pretty positive effect on that. Dairy protein is is actually a pretty good source of protein, quite honestly. But again: If tolerated!

When we're looking at muscle gain: Obviously, you gotta hit your protein goals. Muscle is made out of protein, the literature is quite clear on that - and that carbohydrates are not required for muscle synthesis. What we require for muscle protein synthesis is adequate protein, adequate leucine - which you will undoubtedly get on a meat-based diet.

We know that leucine will stimulate something called mTOR, the mammalian target of rapamycin, which is involved in anabolism. The minimum effective dose for that seems to be 2.5 to 3 grams per meal. And we can stimulate that at a frequency of about three to four hours.

Unfortunately some of that research is based upon whey protein which is pretty rapidly absorbed. So I don't know if that three to four hour... if those those numbers hold up on a carnivore diet. But based on what we know from the other research, that's what we're looking at.

Post workout protein: One or two hours within a workout seems to be helpful. So eating a steak within a couple of hours of training, if your goal is to put on muscle.

Then the other thing that's important - and this is where carbohydrates can become helpful - is a caloric surplus.

As I stated, meat and fat is particularly satiating, and therefore a caloric surplus can be difficult to get into. Some people might require to eat 4, 5, 6 pounds of meat a day, which can be difficult to get you into a sufficient caloric surplus, to build muscle.

We know that carbohydrates can help to restore glycogen stores, although eating enough protein generally does that as well. What we're seeing is you can put on muscle, but it requires effort and work. Then obviously, you've got to do the training that goes with that.

Fat loss, a fun topics for me:

FAT LOSS

- Step 1 -deal with food addiction!!!!
  - Physiology- Satiety, Nutrient sufficiency
  - Psychology- stress, entertainment, boredom, comfort, family/peer pressure
  - CHANGE RELATIONSHIP WITH FOOD
- DIETS FAIL when hunger is constant or food is not tolerated/palatable
- Satiating food
- External support- family, community, coaching

Because it's very controversial, and there's so many people that get wound up about what's the best way to lose fat. The answer is: There are a number of ways. But within the context of a carnivore diet...

I always ask people a bunch of questions when they're dealing with fat loss, particularly if they have food addiction issues. With many people, the reason they gained a lot of weight, is because they couldn't stop eating the garbage food. They couldn't stop eating the cookies, the cakes, the pizzas, the food that tends to be a problem.

And most people can't eat a small amount of this. We know that, we've got the potato chip commercials saying *bet you can't just eat one!* They're right, you can't! So you have to deal with that addiction behavior.

The first goal whenever I'm taking care of clients or discussing this with people, I say "You must deal with the food addiction issues!" You've got to figure out how to keep them from relapsing, ending up face down in a bowl of ice cream or a plate of cupcakes.

I think there's a physiologic aspect to that, and we talked about satiety. There are hormones that are responsive to the nutrition that we eat. Cholecystokinin is particularly responsive to protein and fat, that is one of our satiety

86

hormones. It's named because it makes our gallbladder contract. It's a pretty important satiety hormone.

There's mechanical satiety: When you stretch your gut out with high fiber, high volume food. This is why some of the plant-based options that are high volume do work. But that often ends up with people having a number of GI difficulties. Whether it's just acute things, like bloating, gas, pain, constipation - or long-term issues, where they develop IBS.

So satiety, again, is important. And you have to have nutrient sufficiency. It doesn't do you any good eating a high calorie diet if you're missing some key nutrients. An animal-based diet tends to be very high in nutrition, very high in bioavailable nutrients.

Then you have to deal with the psychological aspect of this. Whether you eat for stress, entertainment, boredom, comfort, family pressure or peer pressure.

The environment that we are in will not change! We're not going to wake up tomorrow and all of a sudden all the junk food is going to disappear from the earth. The TV commercials imploring you to eat the latest junk food.

And your family members trying to tell you *eat another bite,* that's never going to go away. So you have to be able to deal with the psychological aspects of it. It's much easier when the physiology is in place. You've got to change your relationship with food, I think this is the number one step here.

Diets will fail when hunger is constant, or food is not tolerated or palatable. If you want a prescription for failing on a diet, tell somebody be hungry all the time or tell someone to eat food they don't like. I mean, that's a guaranteed recipe for something thst's not going to work. The food needs to be satiating.

And I think you need to have some degree of external support, for most people. Whether it's family, community coaching - that's some of the stuff that we try to provide at MeatRX for people doing a carnivore-based diet.

Because a lot of people just don't get support. A lot of times... if you're a meat-eater these days, you're almost considered a pariah. You're kind of going the way of the smoker, we're gonna start demonizing meat eaters, which hopefully we don't get to.

Fat loss approaches:

FAT LOSS

- High Fat Approach
- This can provide profound satiety and can often be hypo-caloric
- Nutritional Ketosis often results
- Some note improved cognition, better mood etc..
- Often works with food addicts, significantly obese (IF IT CAUSES SATIETY)
- Fat sources important

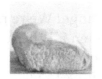 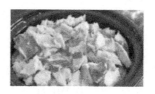

The high fat approach, this can provide profound satiety - and can often be hypocaloric! That is to say people will get so satiated from eating a very high fat diet that they end up eating a hypocaloric diet. What does that mean? Well, a hypocaloric diet means you're losing weight.

I don't want to get too much into the different metabolic advantages. But by definition, if you're losing weight you are eating less calories than you need to maintain weight. So you might eat a lot of calories but you still may be relatively hypocaloric.

Nutritional ketosis often results from this. Some will note other added benefits like improved cognition, better mood, et cetera. This often is a good approach for people that are food addicts or significantly obese - with the caveat that if it causes satiety. And the fat sources are important.

I've got pictured here some cut up beef fat that I talked about, some egg yolks, that's some wagyu beef - which is not in everyone's budget. But certainly, it's nice if you can get it.

If you are eating a bunch of dairy fat and you're throwing stevia in there, so you make some heavy cream and you whip it up, throw a bunch of stevia in there - you're going to be able to overeat much more easily.

So again, if you are a food addict and you're eating fat to a point where you overeat it, then this approach may not work for you. But for most people it does seem to work pretty well.

There's a high protein approach:

FAT LOSS

- High Protein Approach
- Need to be no longer dealing with food addiction
- Works for getting very lean (athletes, physique competitors)
- Lean meats, with periodic high fat re-feeds (3-7 days)
- Possibly more hunger, need to time meals to deal with hunger (Grehlin diurnal variation)
- Protein often 70+%
- Not a long term sustainable strategy
- Fat re-feed not a gorge session

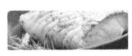

I've used all these approaches myself, personally. I think you need to be out of that phase of being a food addict. If you're dealing with food addiction then this is not the best approach for you.

It works very well for getting very lean: Athletes, physique competitors, these are often people that need to, or want to be, at a level of body fat that is, quite honestly, not physiologically normal. These are the people that are quite 'shredded', or down sub 10% body fat for males and sub 15% body fat for females.

The way I approach this and the way I deal with people that want to do that is: We work on basically lean meats with periodic high fat refeeds, and these occur about every 3 to 7 days. The reason for that is

- fat is critically important for our health in general, but
- it also it helps with compliance, and
- it helps with maintaining metabolic rates.

There probably and possibly will be more hunger to deal with on this approach! You need to time your meals to deal with hunger.

Some of you guys are aware of ghrelin, it is a hormone that stimulates our hunger. It is a hormone that's primarily secreted from our upper GI tract, but there are several locations in our body that secrete ghrelin.

Ghrelin tends to peak in a diurnal fashion, with the majority of it occurring later in the day. That's why often in people who wake up in the morning, they're not hungry - but come evening time, many people are dealing with hunger. So timing the meals to deal with ghrelin can be helpful.

Protein, in this case, can often be as high as 70 percent! And believe me, that's hard to do when you're eating a meat based diet.

You have to eat particularly lean cuts of meat, things like fish, shrimp, those things are important. And I still recommend getting some red meat in the diet on a daily basis. So you have to go with very lean cuts of red meat when you're doing this.

This, in my view, is not a long-term sustainable strategy. This helps for getting down to a certain level of leanness, and then you have to figure out what you're going to do to sustain that. I've seen that if you can sustain a certain level of leanness for about six months, then you kind of reach a new set point, where you can maintain that a little bit easier.

And then the fat refeeds - occurring 3 three to 7 days - are not gorge sessions! It's not a cheat day to just eat as much as you possibly can. I did that initially when I was trying that...

and failed miserably! Because I just was eating something like 7000, 8000 calories in fat. And at that time I was including dairy fat.

Again, I don't think dairy fat is a particularly good thing to refeed on. Staying with the other source of that we talked about is going to work better. But this is where you bring the ribeye steaks back in, the short ribs and the skirt steaks... which is delicious, by the way.

All right. Some considerations that I've seen in the carnivore community, particularly when it comes to fat loss:

CONSIDERATIONS

- Men tend to get results faster
- Men may respond better to satiating effects of CCK vs women
- Most women seem to prefer higher fat approach
- Resistance training is a very important confounder
- Age and digestive function make alter protein availibilty/needs

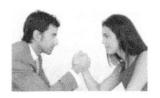

Now, men tend to get results faster, sorry ladies. Particularly women that are in that perimenopausal time, it's harder for women. That's just the way it is.

There is a study out there looking at CCK (Cholecystokinin) and saw that its satiating effect was better on men than women, and then also children, in that study. So that may be part of the reason most women tend to, in my experience, prefer the higher fat approach.

Resistance training: If you're working out, strength training, it seems to be a confounder which may drive you one way or the other. Often people that include more resistance training in their diet do tend to skew more towards a higher protein strategy.

Age and digestive function may alter protein availability and needs. What I mean by that is: As we get older, particularly as we get older, we start to accumulate disease. I think one of those diseases is a decreased function of our digestive tract.

Maybe a decreased ability to secrete stomach acid, maybe other enzymes, proteases and lipases, and absorptive capacity... just as the digestive tract starts to get worse as we age.

Now, is that a natural consequence of aging, or is that just an accumulation of disease from eating the wrong diet, poor lifestyle? Probably more likely than not, it has to do with poor lifestyle over time, rather than just flat out age. Typically most people recommend to up your protein as you get older.

Okay. What are some of the expectations? What do I expect to see?

EXPECTATIONS

- Decreases in inflammatory markers (hs CRP)
- Decreased Triglycerides
- Decreased glucose and glycemic variability
- Decreased blood pressure
- Decreased NAFLD/Visceral fat
- Increased HDL
- Increased BUN, Creatinine (particularly with HP approach)
- Variable effect on LDL, TC

This isn't a comprehensive list, but in general these tend to be true:

We see a decrease in inflammatory markers, such as high sensitivity c-reactive protein. We see a decrease in triglycerides, we see decreased glucose and glycemic variability. We see a decrease in blood pressure, we see decreases in visceral fat, including non-alcoholic fatty liver disease.

We see increased HDL, we see increases in blood urea nitrogen and creatinine, particularly with a high protein approach. And the effect on LDL and total cholesterol is variable. Many people will see significant increases, some people see no change, some people will see it actually go down.

And some of these are things we'd like to test in our clinical trial, just to confirm that. But that is what I'm seeing on a daily basis, with frequent feedback from the community.

All right, some odds and ends:

ODD AND ENDS

- Cystatin C is a better test to assess renal function in carnivores (not confounded by dietary protein intake)
- Gout may flare up initially, but generally resolves as metabolic syndrome/systemic inflammation improves
- Those undergoing chemotherapy for cancer note better tolerance with a carnivorous diet
- Previous cholecystectomy is not a contraindication to diet

Cystatin c... I don't know how many folks are health care providers in here. But: If you're testing someone and you want to assess renal function in carnivores, particularly those on a high protein diet, cystatin c is a far better test than your standard serum creatinine level, and the estimated glomerular filtration rate that is based upon that calculation.

That is to say: We know that creatinine will often be elevated in people on a high protein diet. And we know that that number is used to calculate the GFR (the glomerular filtration rate) - so that can give you an artificially increased creatinine and an artificially decreased GFR, confounded by protein intake.

So if you look at cystatin c, you will take that confounder out and you'll get a better assessment of what the actual renal function is.

Basically every person that I've seen, that's been on a carnivore diet, has been concerned about that, or the doctor's been concerned about that. We say that assessing cystatin c... it almost always invariably turns out good, it shows that they have normal, and very good, renal function.

Gout, I get a lot of questions on gout. Gout may flare up initially, particularly if you're at risk for gout or you already have gout. And those people that are at risk for gout are the people that are at risk for diabetes, those people that have metabolic syndromes.

With people that are metabolically unhealthy, obese, high levels of visceral fat, you may see a flare up.

But generally - as time goes by, as those metabolic issues resolve, systemic inflammation improves - we see gout go away, despite even elevated levels of uric acid, which may occur.

I'll just touch on cancer, I know it's a controversial topic. But we have a number of people that are dealing with cancer, treating cancer.

As we know, many people use ketogenic diets as an adjuvant for cancer treatments. What I'm seeing is people that are going through cancer treatment with a carnivore diet seem to have much better tolerance to the treatments, whether it's chemotherapy or radiation.

They don't seem to get as sick, they don't seem to have some of the profound vomiting and things like that, that often go with chemotherapy. So that's at least something that can be used as a beneficial part.

Does it prevent cancer, improve cancer outcomes? You can't say that yet. I don't think we have any data, particularly on a carnivore diet, that would prove that.

Although Dr. Clemons and Dr. Toth in Hungary are doing that research and they're getting some data in that regard, particularly with regard to brain tumors.

If you've had a previous cholecystectomy or you've had your gallbladder out, it is *not* a contraindication to this diet. We see that with... again, with all kinds of low carb diets:

Most of the people that lost their gallbladder lost it before they went on a low carb diet. In fact, many people argue that the standard american high carb junk food diet is what's driving the high cholecystectomy rate in the population.

You certainly can go on a high fat carnivore diet long term, without a gallbladder. Now, there may be some adjustments that you might do. Some people find that adding some digestive supplements early on can be helpful.

We do seem to see that the common bile duct which is left, becomes a reservoir for bile, and you can get a bolus of bile... which is what the gallbladder does:

It squeezes when we eat a high fat meal to secrete bile into the small intestine, which breaks up the fat, emulsifies it like a detergent - so it can be more readily acted upon by digestive enzymes, like lipases, and then later absorbed. So you can do it with a cholistectomy.

Okay, I think that's all I've got. I'm going to open it up for questions!

Question:
Joe Rogan said a carnivore diet causes aggression and diarrhea, are these common side effects?

Answer:
So aggression... I don't know. I mean, some people feel more energized and they want to work out harder. I haven't seen like violent aggression, but I think he's talking about just a desire to use the body in a physical fashion. I don't know if it's the same as violent aggression.

But I think you just feel like you're just more energized and you want to do things.

As far as diarrhea is concerned, it seems to occur in about a quarter of the population that do this. There's a couple things going on: For some people, particularly when they go high fat and they're not used to it, they end up exceeding their absorptive capacity for fat - so they'll get steatoria, which is fat in the stool.

That often occurs for a couple weeks. Some people find that either adjusting the fat down - or up, in some cases - can help with that.

What we do know is the colon is presented with a very different situation on a carnivore diet, than it is when we're on a high carbohydrate, high fiber diet. Because one of the roles of the colon is to absorb fluid and electrolytes. So when we ingest all this fluid and electrolyte rather than wasting it all, our colon will reabsorb that to save that - and so the minerals are very important.

But when we're on a high fiber diet, much of that fluid and electrolyte is trapped within the fiber. So the colon is not faced with that. So when we eliminate the fiber, now the only thing that exits the small intestine is all purely liquid based.

We know that from looking at patients with ileostomies. They no longer have solid material in the small intestines, it's all liquid. So sometimes that little liquid overwhelms the current capacity of the colon to reabsorb that high fluids coming from the small intestine. And so it takes time for that to adapt.

Usually, this is an adaptation process. But there are some things:

Maybe too much fat. Some people have issues with eggs, some people have issues with different cuts of meat. I've seen pork being an issue.

High amounts of spices, if you're eating a lot of spicy food, that can be an irritant to the GI system - and the body is trying to get rid of it quickly.

I would say, in about 25% of the people, that occurs. It tends to be short-lived. People with underlying bowel issues like IBS, this may last for longer, just because that's a primary gut issue which takes longer to heal.

Question:

My butcher here in spain says that fat, especially around the organs, are high in toxins. He gives me grease whenever I ask for that. Is there merit to this?

Answer:

I think that's a theoretical concern as to how much toxins there are. Certainly, in humans we store things that are fat soluble in our fat. How much that affects an actual human by ingesting it? That is really purely speculative. I have not seen any human data...

The bottom line is, there are just not any human trials on this stuff. This is why it's important to do those human trials. So anybody that's going to say that, it's purely speculation.

Typically, when we look at things like glyphosate... which is an active ingredient in roundup: When we see what actually ends up in animal fat or animal tissues, it is such a miniscule, tiny amount that it is really, really not an issue. So, eating fat is not an issue in my view, regardless of the animal, for the most part.

I know it's controversial. But people that are sort of bringing that argument up are basically purely speculative. There's no human data that would confirm that. Do we need to do these trials that would test that? Absolutely, I'd agree!

But I have not seen anything that would confirm that. And again, I'm looking at results in human beings and that's what I have to go on. So if you feel that that's a concern and you're worried about it, there's probably a thousand other more important things in the environment to worry about.

Question:

Do people with liver disease need to avoid the carnivore diet?

Answer:

In general, no. It depends on what the liver disease is. If you're having issues with high levels of ammonia production, then you're going to have to limit your protein content. But for the average person with... and liver disease is a broad category.

The most common liver disease that we see is *non-alcoholic fatty liver disease.* And my experience is, that this diet generally improves that.

Now, the caveat to this is: If you are overeating on any diet, in my view, then that can be a problem for your liver. But meat by itself eaten in a in a way that provides satiety and doesn't lead to weight gain is fine for the liver.

Question:
I told my optometrist, cardiologist about the carnivore diet, she said I will get cataracts.

Answer:
I don't know of any data that would show that eating a meat diet would cause cataracts. In fact, we have an optometrist, cardiologist, that has seen the exact opposite occur.

Interesting topic: We just had a person in our group this morning, said her glaucoma, her eye pressures went from 22 to 17, taking her from basically glaucoma to non-glaucoma.

And the optometrists have seen improvements in cataracts, with the carnivore diet.

Question:
Is this a long-term eating style or only temporary to accomplish a goal?

Answer:
Both! I mean, some people have done it long term. I've been doing it for 4 years, people are doing it for 20+ years. Many people use it as a tool, a short-term tool. You do what works.

I would tell anybody: If the diet no longer works for you, you should quit the diet! If it's working for you long-term, you enjoy it and you have a good quality of life... then you do it for as long as you need to. Just be cognizant of potential issues and monitor for those.

But many people use it for a short term way to solve problems. If we use it as an elimination diet, it works very, very well. It's very effective at helping you solve problems.

When we're playing the elimination game... when you have one variable, it's a lot easier than when you have 20 things you're trying to deal with, figuring out what the problem is.

Question:
Does this way of eating have positive effects on people with thyroid issues? Getting the numbers within normal range?

Answer:
It can, and it has! I've seen people with things like Hashimoto's and other types of hypothyroidism significantly improve their clinical symptoms, which is a number one concern.

But we also see normalization of things, particularly TSA. We do know that with low carb diets, often people will run low levels of T3... which many people think is a normal physiologic adaptation to the low carb state.

Just analogous to low insulin. Like, we see with a low carb diet, many people have low insulin, relative to what is normal. The normal range of fasting insulin in this country is about 8, whereas a lot of people on low carb and carnivore diets see their insulin levels drop below 5, and often below 3!

Everybody's excited about that because then we know we're insulin sensitive. We also see a situation where we become *thyroid sensitive*. That is why we may see lower levels of T3, despite normal clinical function. Again, clinical function is - at the end of the day - what we're all concerned about.

Question:
Would the lean approach with fat refeed days work well for pregnant or menopausal women?

Answer:
It can, it certainly can. I've seen people that have done that.

Question:
As a carnivore, how many grams of protein do you eat on average per day?

Answer:
It depends. I have eaten as much as 600 grams in a day, to as little as a 100 grams. So it really depends on what I'm doing. But oin general, as an athlete, I tend to shoot for about a gram per pound, but that varies.

Question:
What is the most effective way for women to lose body fat in the beginning of menopause?

Answer:
Goodness! I think there's a lot of things that are going there. I think resistance training is important. Managing your satiety... again, when I talked about why are we obese in the first place: Fixing the food addiction issue has to be the first goal there.

Getting adequate protein and adjusting your protein to your activity levels is important. I think protein is an incredibly important macronutrient. But satiety is going to be... whatever's going to give you satiety, really, that's going to be it. Whether it's high fat or high protein.

But, including some resistance training in there is probably the general successful way.

I think I've got all the questions.

Other Host Andy Schreiber:
Listen, thank you so much Dr. Baker! That was great, I really appreciate it. I hope you had a good time, too.

Dr. Baker:
Thank you Andy!

Schreiber:
All right, thank you so much!

Other Summary Books

25% of the royalties of this book will be donated to Dr. Seyfrieds research!

This research will actually make a REAL impact, as it studies the real causes and treatment opportunities of cancer!

This book is a summary of Dr. Thomas Seyfrieds book "Cancer as a metabolic disease" and comprises transcripts of his talks and interviews, as well as texts by his collegue Dr. Dominic D'Agostiono and Travis Christofferson (whose foundation will be supported by this book).

Here the original Book description:

The book addresses controversies related to the origins of cancer and provides solutions to cancer management and prevention. It expands upon Otto Warburg's well-known theory that all cancer is a disease of energy metabolism. However, Warburg did not link his theory to the "hallmarks of cancer" and thus his theory was discredited.

This book aims to provide evidence, through case studies, that cancer is primarily a metabolic disease requring metabolic solutions for its management and prevention.

Support for this position is derived from critical assessment of current cancer theories. Brain cancer case studies are presented as a proof of principle for metabolic solutions to disease management, but similarities are drawn to other types of cancer, including breast and colon, due to the same cellular mutations that they demonstrate.

THE CARNIVORE DIET
OF
DR JORDAN PETERSON
& MIKHAILA PETERSON

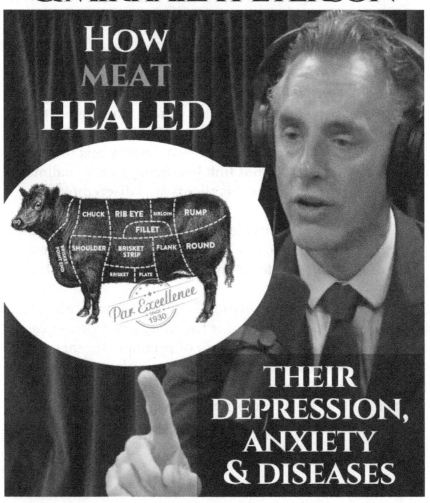

HOW MEAT HEALED

THEIR DEPRESSION, ANXIETY & DISEASES

The book offers 11 Chapters of revised transcripts of Dr. Jordan Peterson & Mikhaila Peterson on:

- how they cured their disease, depression and health issues with the carnivore diet and
- how ill people could start this kind of eating as well.

The Transcripts are as follows:

1. The Agenda with Steve Paikin Digesting Depression
2. Joe Rogan Podcast 1070
3. Joe Rogan Podcast 1139
4. Podcast Interview of Mikhaila Peterson with Robb Wolf, including blood work
5. Podcast Interview with Ivor Cummins
6. Talk by Mikhaila Peterson at the Carnivore Conference in Boulder, 2019
7. Mikhaila Petersons Blog: The Diet Introduction of her Lion Diet on YouTube
8. Mikhaila Peterson: Should you start an elimination diet?
9. Mikhaila Peterson: Jordan Peterson's Lion Diet
10 Mikhaila Peterson: The Lion Diet (Introduction of her diet on YouTube

11. Bonus-Transcript: Dr. Shawn Baker talking about his coronary calcium score and overall health status with years of being carnivore.

The transcriptions are revised, which means that the grammar and the wordsequences got corrected, adding phrases here and there, as well as leaving out other elements that hinder understanding and the joy of reading.

Sources

Chapter

1)   Text (editors revised transcription) based on Youtube video:

Channel: Tom Bilyeu

Channel-Url:
https://www.youtube.com/channel/UCnYMOamNKLGVlJgRUbamveA

Title: The Evolutionary Logic Behind the Carnivore Diet | Shawn Baker on Health Theory

Video-Url: https://www.youtube.com/watch?v=wrfVoL_7kA4

2)   Text and slides based on Youtube video:

Channel: KetoCon

Channel-Url:
https://www.youtube.com/channel/UC2mNCHWMsOFsieQuw4jdZTQ

Title: Dr Shawn Baker Nutrition, Exercise, and Healthcare

Video-Url: https://www.youtube.com/watch?v=lEq1xMaGhyw

3)   Text and slides based on Youtube video:

Channel: NSNG Foods

Channel-Url:
https://www.youtube.com/channel/UCI84sQaJ6IHb4BAYcMVNQgA

Title: Tailoring the Carnivore Diet for Specific Goals with Dr. Shawn Baker - NSNG Summit 2020

Video-Url: https://www.youtube.com/watch?v=Jh43YFwvXro

Thanks to Dr. Shawn Baker for his important work to cure people of our modern diseases!

His website: https://shawn-baker.com/

His Community website: https://revero.com/
(former MeatRX.com)

His YouTube Channel:

https://www.youtube.com/c/ShawnBakerMD

_____

Version 1.0   5. October 2021

_____

Made in the USA
Las Vegas, NV
25 April 2024

89146740R00059